What I Wish My Patients Knew..

A Behind the Scenes Look at Primary Care and How to Survive as a Patient

Amy Fitzgerald Pelloquin M.D.

What I Wish My Patients Knew

Copyright ©2024 by Amy Fitzgerald Pelloquin

All rights reserved.

Printed in the United States of America. No part of this book may be used or reproduced in any manner whatsoever without written permission from the author(s).

Layout and Design: Variance Author Services

www.varianceauthorservices.com

What I Wish My Patients Knew..

A Behind the Scenes Look at Primary Care and How to Survive as a Patient

Amy Fitzgerald Pelloquin M.D.

DEDICATED TO:

MY FELLOW HEALTH CARE WORKERS: FOR CONTINUING TO CARE DESPITE IT ALL.

AND TO MARY JANE, WHO ENDED EVERY APPOINTMENT WITH A SMILE AND A HUG NO MATTER THE CHALLENGE.

A deep thank you:

To my family, especially my husband who continues his work so I can explore.

To my heart-sisters: the gift I never thought to ask for.

Table of Contents

Introduction 1

Chapter 1
From There to Here
(AKA: What the heck happened?!) 9

Chapter 2
The Patient Perspective
(AKA: I hate feeling vulnerable
and disempowered!) 21

Chapter 3
The Changing Reality of Healthcare
(AKA: What the hell happened to Marcus Welby? You younger guys will have to look this up.) 26

Chapter 4
Scheduling and Appointments
(AKA: Just how long can I wait on hold, and can you please get some better music?) 32

Chapter 5
Understanding and Selecting a Provider

(AKA: Where did all the cowboys, I mean primary care providers go?) 59

Chapter 6:
Medications
(AKA: Why didn't you send my prescription in?) 78

Chapter 7
Specialty Referrals (Consultations)
(AKA: If you don't know, send me to someone who does!) 119

Chapter 8
Lab Results/Imaging/Procedures
(AKA Do I really need this test?!) 134

Chapter 9
Testing Results
(AKA: I saw my results! Am I dying?!) 150

Chapter 10
Paperwork
(AKA: The bane of everyone's existence) 162

Chapter 11
Electronic Health Records (EHR or EMR)
(AKA: This was supposed to make things easier- what the hell happened?) 16

CHAPTER 12
PROVIDER "GRADING"
(AKA: THERE IS NO STUDYING FOR THIS TEST!) 179

CHAPTER 13
INSURANCE
(AKA: DO I NEED A COLLEGE DEGREE TO INTERPRET THIS? OR... I HAVE A COLLEGE DEGREE AND STILL DON'T UNDERSTAND THIS!) 189

CHAPTER 14
AGING, END OF LIFE ISSUES AND DEATH
(AKA: LET'S NOT TALK ABOUT THAT....) 200

CHAPTER 15
THE PERSONAL ACCOUNTABILITY FACTOR
(AKA: AT LEAST HALF OF THIS IS ON YOU!) 218

CHAPTER 16
THE DISCONNECT
(AKA: THIS ISN'T FREAKING WORKING.) 227

CHAPTER 17
REFLECTIONS ON HEALTH
(AKA: OUTSIDE THE BOX IS NOT ALWAYS A BAD PLACE TO BE!) 239

CHAPTER 18
FOOD FOR THOUGHT
(AKA: IS THE GLASS HALF FULL OR HALF EMPTY?) 250

APPENDIX A 260

ABOUT THE AUTHOR 279

Introduction

I stood in line with a pounding heart and sweating hands as I waited with my medical school class for my turn to receive that coveted white coat. A symbol of so much hard work, knowledge, responsibility, ego and power. And these were just the *"short"* white coats of a medical student when you were deemed safe enough to interact and touch patients. The *"long"* white coats were the ultimate reward but there was no ceremony around that initiation; just the plastic bag handed to you with your coat inside. No fanfare, but a deep sense of pride and accomplishment in my name and M.D. so blatantly embroidered above the pocket. It felt like a benediction to put that long white coat on for the first time. Then, the reality and terror of that awesome responsibility set in.

These memories are so vivid that it is difficult to believe that it has now been over 30 years since I received that first white coat. Many years as a physician, and a career colored with a remarkably diverse background of experiences. First, at an academic institution instructing medical students and residents, then in the hospital taking care of acutely ill patients and ultimately in outpatient primary care clinics. I have seen the various faces of the economics behind healthcare: the issues that an academic institution has, those that occur with a physician owned clinic, and those found within large corporate entities running the show. Each of these experiences provided a vastly different and distinct view of how the healthcare system operates from the perspective of an internal medicine physician. I realize in retrospect that I had navigated the majority of these with the map of my initial training within the halls of academia, where traditional science was the only accepted truth. I thought that this well-defined and time-honored structure was the end all and be all of how medicine was supposed to work. But what a constricting space! It was an interesting journey over the ensuing years as I slowly developed an awareness that there is much that didn't fit into this rigid model. But I kept my head down and continued to do my work in the way that I had been taught. I mean, all those distinguished professors couldn't be wrong, could they? The edges began to fray around my dedication to what I had been taught the longer I worked though. I felt the beginnings of slight panic emerge as I embraced the full scope of my disenchantment. Had I really spent countless hours studying, at bedsides, reviewing radiology films and labs, taking certification exams to prove my worth to just change careers? I had felt called to this profession at a young age, so to just stop was unthinkable.

About the time I was reaching a crisis point, I happened to run into an emergency department physician that I was friends with but hadn't spoken to in over a year. Her face was glowing as she told me about an Integrative Medicine fellowship she was taking with the University of Arizona. Aha! That's what I wanted; that look of passion that I saw on her face. It took about 5 minutes for me to look up information on that fellowship, but a few more weeks to convince myself that it was ok to question, ok to explore. I finally took the plunge, and two years and many hours and late nights later, I entered the world of Integrative Medicine. Finally, I thought here is what I've been searching for. And yes, this did fill in some of those gaps that I had noticed quite nicely, but there were still weak spots in the foundation of the care that I was providing to my patients daily. The fellowship had managed to reignite my passion about medicine but still didn't provide all of the answers. Unlike before the fellowship however, there was no angst about moving forward and exploring what would provide more answers. It was like the tight boundaries that had been placed (or had I placed them?)

on me had dissolved. So, I kept searching, and stumbled upon a spiritual path of all things. For a girl raised in a strict Southern Baptist family, this was a huge step for me. I was shocked to find there were a lot of ingrained beliefs (ones that I hadn't realized I had) now being challenged. Ironically, as opposed to providing the answers that I was so desperately seeking, this pursuit just raised more questions. The most worrisome thing is that it specifically prompted me to evaluate just exactly what is healing. More and more questions now, not less.

I finally realized and acknowledged there is just not an answer to every question in medicine. A hard pill to swallow when I spent years training to learn the answer to whatever question that my patients asked. What I did learn is I don't need all the answers but I need to ask the right questions, both of my patients and myself. The biggest one I came to during this process was *"Am I helping patients heal or helping to support a system that at its core is focused on sustaining illness, not preventing it?"* What an uncomfortable position to be in, and I thought after all this seeking and work how I had arrived right back to this place of disillusionment. What now? How to manage? What to actually do with all of this knowledge and awareness? Well, I withdrew from participating in our current system as a primary care physician as it seemed too inadequate to try to change things from that position. The first couple of months after I ended my practice, I sat in a chair on my back deck and looked at the mountains for hours, healing from the many previously unrecognized emotional wounds created by the stress of working in such a broken system. I began to realize at a deeper level the toll that I and my various health care worker colleagues pay to care for our patients within the construct of modern healthcare in the U.S. As more and more is heaped onto the outdated ship that is our current medical system, we took on the responsibility of filling in all the holes in the hull that appeared. Too many captains running a ship with no knowledge of how the ship runs, and not enough crew. For a time, I wanted nothing more to do with any of it and finally gave myself the freedom to consider a completely different path. However, as the days turned into months, the reason that I began my journey back as a teenager began to resurface, and I slowly felt my passion to help people reignite stronger than ever but changed. I began to reflect on ways to help in a broader context. I thought of what I could do and how that would look to help create a better system for patients and providers, but felt overwhelmed at the immensity of what needed to change. Then I remembered, I don't have to change the system from the top down, I can work from the bottom up. I can help all the players on the front lines from both sides to understand the other. So much frustration and anger on both sides and often directed at the perceived other side – I think because we all feel so disempowered. I considered what an empowered patient who understood the system better could bring to the table in effecting change that benefits not only them, but the providers and the entire system. We as patients and providers are so much more powerful as a team, and somehow that seems to have been lost in most primary care clinics. I hope these pages offer you as patients a peek behind the curtain to the mechanics of what it takes to provide your care in our current system, and to us as providers, reminding us that the knowledge of these issues we take for granted most of our patients don't know. Knowledge is a type of power and the more you know the more empowered you are.

Chapter 1
From There to Here
(AKA: What the heck happened?!)

As a medical student I firmly believed that life was to be conquered with rules and structure. If you study hard, get an "A," then good things will happen and you will be successful. You simply go from point "A" to "B" and then get to "C." My years of college and medical school reinforced this completely. It was a simple process and I didn't understand why other students that I knew made it so hard. Just follow the rules! Don't go out and party the night before a test, take notes and read them over and over until 3 am and you have them memorized, and make sure that your life revolves around your work.

At the same time, a part of me knew that there was another piece to all of this and it was there, flowing underneath at all times, asking to be remembered. I was an artist when I was younger and deeply understood that the best paintings aren't produced with a linear, logical, algorithm. They spring from that creative side of us that can see the infinite whole. But, the rigid demands of science, which is based on finite defined boundaries, paired with an era where logic and the left brain were valued above all else proved to be more powerful. The role of *"competing with the boys"* I played so often that it became who I thought I was. I remember, during one of my first days of medical school orientation, a speaker who passionately spoke about the importance of living in the moment, having compassion and occasionally taking the long route to work; you might see a newborn foal playing in a field as he had. He was a psychologist but with his beard, hiking pants, casual shirt and such an open display of *"feelings"* he was nothing more than a hippie holdover to be discounted and ridiculed. I didn't want any of that. I wanted the white coat and the prestige and power that went with it. Me and my class's reaction reinforced how unimportant we thought his ideas were, and that vulnerability and compassion were things to be hidden away as signs of weakness. I remember that we mocked his gestures and sayings for weeks after school began, and especially when the pressure became more intense. It is interesting in retrospect that we did this. He must have triggered others besides me with his comments about vulnerability. Funny that all these years later I cannot remember a single other speaker during orientation but his presentation remains vividly clear in my memory. When I returned for my 30-year medical school reunion and visited the classroom where I spent so many hours, I didn't see all the accomplished lecturers who had provided such a wealth of knowledge. What I saw was this goofy psychologist standing down and to the left pleading with us to be more human. Perhaps my subconscious knew what was truly important even then and held tight to this memory for me.

So, if these human qualities weren't important to me, what was? Knowledge. My patients have always received the best knowledge that I could provide them. I read my journals, kept up my CME (continuing medical education), attended conferences and basically checked all the boxes to stay current in primary care. I could never learn enough. I thought this was the way to provide the very best possible care and worked hard to share all of it with my patients (in retrospect, whether they wanted to hear it or not). I ran from room to room with a brisk pace and threw open the exam door ready to do battle on their behalf, armed with guidelines, data and lots of recommendations (or were they just mandates?). I knew exactly what they should do and what they shouldn't do. I needed to share all of this knowledge that I had and force them to comply. After all, this was the paternalistic method of medicine that had been ingrained into me for years. I laugh now, as I know that while this knowledge is critically important, it has only been in the relatively recent past that I have come to understand the deep value of those qualities that I once pushed aside. When we are sick, we do need the most up to date interventions that medicine has to offer and an informed provider, AND we also need the system that is providing it to reassure us, bolster us and sometimes hold our hands.

When I was in the delivery room with my first daughter, I had the typical *"if it could go wrong, it did go wrong"* scenario. I was very grateful for my obstetrician and her medical expertise and guidance, but I also remember with great detail the curly-haired nurse Elizabeth, who wiped my brow and cared for me with such kindness. She walked with me through that ordeal and actually did hold my hand and spoke words of encouragement while I was at my most vulnerable; she was always there with just the right touch or word. It was as important in that experience for me as anything else that occurred. Looking back, she helped me integrate the experience in such a way that it did not result in the anxiety and trauma it could have. I can recount the tale, but not relive it thanks to her. She listened to what I as her patient needed and acted on that, not working down an algorithm of what I was supposed to need.

- We need more providers who will allow themselves to be open and listen to what their patients actually need as opposed to only what the system thinks their patient needs.
- We need providers who will still listen to their intuition as well as the algorithm for a condition.

I worry that as patients and providers become more important as data points on a spreadsheet these qualities will continue to fall by the wayside. Our current healthcare system becomes more difficult to navigate with each passing day. I ask that you consider compassion for the patients trying to find their way, for the providers struggling to juggle the demands of a system that does not value much other than the bottom line, and hope what you find in this book helps you, even if only in some small way, in accomplishing this difficult ask.

Chapter 1A:

In this book you will hear me refer to providers, patients and "the system." We know who the patients are, that's me and you. Basically, all of us at some point will be patients. The providers referred to are a composite of doctors and mid-level providers such as nurse practitioners and physician assistants. But this term can include nurses, medical assistants, physical therapists, respiratory therapists and others on the front line of patient care. To go even further, in many ways it can also include administrative personnel such as the front desk staff ~~personnel~~ at the health care facilities who interact with patients on a daily basis. Then who is *"the system"*? According to Merriam Webster *"the system"* is a noun that refers to a *powerful government or social organization that controls people's lives.* This seems particularly appropriate here. It is organizations that control how your health care dollars are actually spent: how many nurses are allotted to care for you during your hospitalization, which medication you have access to through your insurance, how many times you can see a physical therapist each year, which procedure or imaging study you can have, how much time your provider can spend with you, how your provider is paid and on and on. In years past, providers had a large say in the actual "how" your care was planned and implemented. While this made sense to have input from the players actually caring for the patients and interested primarily in each individual patient's outcome, it was often *not economically optimal.* Providers, while intelligent enough to go through rigorous training and testing to actually become providers, are in general not often as proficient in a financial role. And as with any group of people, there were abuses by providers who chose profit over patients, but these were not the majority in my experience. This lack of financial experience became increasingly clear as providers began to manage larger health care entities as opposed to managing an individual practice. Hence, the stepping in of those with more financial prowess to run these entities. Optimal management includes a shared model where the providers on the front line have AS MUCH input into the creation and implementation of policies as the financial individuals in the organization. Unfortunately, the pendulum has now swung 180 degrees to many, if not most health care entities being run by the financial group only. There are providers on panels, boards, and in higher level positions, but frankly many of these roles have no real power in decision making or are filled by providers who have lost touch with what actually occurs on the front lines. Both views are necessary but our current system is out of balance and care is implemented from a spreadsheet showing numbers and data, not the faces of the people impacted.

We're right back to profit over patients, only more pronounced and on a larger scale. A hard truth that is like some politicians, many of those that create and implement the policies don't hold themselves to those policies. If they did, many of the policies would change.

CHAPTER 1B:

I was asked during the review of this book just who is my target audience? The answer is "everyone". Everyone because all of us at some point will be patients. It doesn't matter whether we are physicians, bakers, lawyers, mechanics, salespeople, stay at home parents, students or retirees. We will all interact with our health care system in some way. For many of us the reality of just how broken our system is will become all too apparent when that occurs. There are helpful tips included here to help you navigate this system better and be more empowered. While they will not be applicable to each and every clinic, they can serve as a reference point to open a dialogue with your provider. In contrast there is also a look into the struggles that your provider encounters daily. If you feel a bit of anger as you read, it is because after many edits, I decided that it may be helpful to let some of that bleed through. Please do not misinterpret this as a lack of compassion or empathy for patients. I have been a patient and I deeply understand the trials and tribulations of that role. Most of us do. I want to allow you to feel a small piece of the heartbreak and frustration of your primary care provider's role. We rarely talk about it with our patients, but primary care peer groups and chat boards contain an unending commentary on the despair that is felt by providers trying to care for their patients. Many say they would never encourage anyone to enter primary care in its current form. A few are thriving, but most aren't. Some burn out and just show up every day and go through the motions, some become bitter and angry, some retire early, some invest their time into alternative ways to provide care, some devote more and more time to make it work at the expense of their families and others give up and take their own lives. It is hard to be a compassionate provider when often you are in as dire need of care as your patient. Many of us are emotionally bleeding out slowly and it often feels as if no one cares: not our patients (who truly just don't know how bad it is) and not the system (who certainly does know). Other countries prioritize primary care with a 70:30 ratio of primary care to specialty care, while the US ratio is almost the exact opposite. This disparity is reflected in the resources allocated by government and insurance systems to each: the lack of support is not just perceived, but real. It's the dirty truth behind current US healthcare.

Chapter 2
The Patient Perspective

(AKA: I hate feeling vulnerable and disempowered!)

I have been a patient. I have spent hours in waiting rooms filled with outdated magazines, uncomfortable chairs and stale coffee. I have been to appointments with my parents, friends and children. I have watched my parents sit by the phone all day waiting for a call back from their clinic that never came. I have also listened to them recount their physician visits, one that I actually attended with them, to someone else and wonder whether we were even at the same appointment. We heard completely different things. I have been asked to reschedule my personal appointments, for which I had taken off work but was late for because of a car wreck, and a train, and because my own clinic ran late. I have shown up for an appointment and been told that I didn't have one and I must have written it down on the wrong day *(although I knew that I didn't)*. I have been to the pharmacy and been told my prescription was never sent when the clinic assured me it had been *(and I watched the medical assistant send the prescription in)*. I have been given the wrong medical test and had to have follow up tests to prove that I was given the wrong test, despite my explanation that the initial test was wrong *(they don't even believe a physician on this!)*. I have spent hours on the phone with an insurance company to explore why they didn't pay for the procedure. I have been talked down to by physicians, ignored by nurses while I waited for my medication in the hospital, hung up on by a pharmacy provider customer representative and, fed up with the health care system as a patient. I will not say that I have not screamed at the insanity of it all. So, believe me when I say that I have been in your shoes as a patient.

I understand the patient perspective AND I have been on the other side as a provider. I understand the complexities of the individual positions and of the relationship between the two. Not many individuals have this perspective. The 2020 US population was 329.5 million and according to the American Medical Association data in the *2020 Physician Specialty Data Report* there were 938,966 active physicians among all specialties. Adding to that 2020 number are 211,280 active nurse practitioners (according to nursingprocess.org) and 148,560 physician assistants[1] Some of these physicians and other providers do not provide direct patient care, and may be interventional only, but we'll include them anyway. So, adding these up to include even nonclinical providers, only approximately 0.4% of the population has this unique perspective of being on both sides of this equation. To narrow this down even more, I am focusing on the primary care perspective. According to the National Center for Health Workforce Analysis, in 2021, there were 268,297 primary care physicians in the U.S. In 2022, there were an estimated 270,660 NPs delivering primary care and 26,455 PAs also working in primary care.2 So the total number of these providers is only 565,412, which represents only approximately 0.17% of the population. This relationship is very unique. Although it is a service that relies on monetary exchange, in its finest form it is a sacred trust, one which has existed for centuries in every culture and goes far beyond monetary value. It has hidden behind many faces in many cultures over recorded history but it is essentially, the same relationship. It is in respect for this trust that I offer you a peek behind the curtain to help you understand the physician/provider perspective from the other side of the exam table in the chaotic world of healthcare. It is such a difficult position as a provider to be the bridge between the system and our patients, and it truly takes quite a toll. This knowledge of experiencing both sides is what has sustained me and allowed me to maintain calm *(most of the time)* when I am personally challenged as a patient once again by the system. It has allowed me to take that deep breath and exhale slowly, releasing the intense desire to throw something at a wall and scream.

References

1. https://www.nccpa.net/wp-content/uploads/2022/04/Statistical-Profile-of-Certified-PAs-2020.pdf accessed 5/30/24.

Chapter 3
The Changing Reality of Healthcare

(AKA: What the hell happened to Marcus Welby? You younger guys will have to look this up.)

My patient, a very pleasant neatly dressed middle-aged woman, greeted me as I entered the exam room, sitting on the edge of her chair with perfect posture and a determined look on her face. She promptly handed me several pages from a women's magazine article on thyroid disease and how she knew this was the cause of her ongoing fatigue, despite her recent normal thyroid tests. This I knew was coming, having been forewarned by my nurse. I sighed internally; another visit spent on a magazine article while the million and one things that I needed to review with her about the labs that we needed to order to monitor her diabetes and cholesterol, the medication refills that I would need to complete all flashed through my mind. How in the world was I going to accomplish all of this in a 15-minute appointment? I won't, I thought. I will just now begin my next patient encounter with someone already annoyed that I'm late and will spend 5 precious minutes of that appointment explaining and defending my tardiness. My mind thought through the rest of my morning, preparing for the worst, and hoping that somewhere on my schedule was a simple sore throat. But as an Internal Medicine physician, like most primary care providers, I knew even a simple sore throat would likely lead to more questions and a full visit. Okay – no lunch again today. I took a deep breath and began the visit, going over the article and trying to fit in the rest and indeed running 10 minutes late. I basically gave her a full lecture on thyroid functioning, her recent labs and why she didn't have low thyroid. At the conclusion, she was adamant that she needed to be on thyroid medication and did not feel heard, and basically told me that she had lost some of her confidence in my competence (hinting at finding another physician). I was frustrated and angry with the entire encounter, which I am more than sure she heard loud and clear. My ego had certainly taken a hit – I mean, I had spent years learning and training which seemed to count for nothing with her. I felt that she didn't want to really hear my recommendations *(or my really good thyroid lecture that my medical students had loved)* and trusted this unknown person who had written this article over me, despite our ongoing relationship over several years. We both left feeling frustrated and that our time had been wasted. In retrospect, I likely missed the mark completely and never asked why she thought she needed to be on thyroid medication, and I suspect there was a deeper underlying issue that I didn't find because I was really not "listening" on all levels. I had already mentally mapped out my discussion before I ever went into that room.

This encounter really did happen and stuck in my mind. The unfortunate truth is that an encounter like this where both parties are left frustrated used to be more of the exception than the rule, but in our current health care system has become more of the norm. There is enough blame on each side for the "why" but the bigger concern is that while the specific scenarios change, this outcome of each being frustrated by feelings of not being heard and a sense of disempowerment have increased. One might think that electronic medical records and all of the advancements in healthcare would have done much to alleviate this type of experience. After all, computers were supposed to give providers more time with their patients, for patients to have access to more information than ever and for providers to have more tests to determine what the problem is. Reality is that the opposite has occurred. Patients are more frustrated with their providers and the system, and provider burnout has never been higher. There is less and less time to actually spend with patients, and of what there is, little time is spent actually communicating. Thus, an ever-increasing pool of angry patients with exorbitant medical bills, and providers with exorbitant stacks of computer work and yes, paperwork. This erosion to the provider/patient relationship has been ongoing for quite some time but was below the radar. So, while Covid was a massive jolt to the health care system, and we blame it for much of where we are currently, it actually uncovered the flimsy house that we had built, on an equally flimsy foundation, that we call modern healthcare.

So, how do we "fix" it? I cringe slightly as I use the word "fix" as we don't all agree on what an optimal healthcare system looks like. What we can all agree on is that it needs to change. Changing healthcare is and will be an ongoing challenge and discussion. There are no easy answers, and where we will be in the future as our population ages and physician and provider numbers decline is a worrisome issue to ponder. As individuals we may feel powerless in the face of this, which leads to even more stress and frustration. As my encounter demonstrated, neither patients nor providers feel heard or respected, and often encounters are adversarial with each side trying to advance their individual agendas. Agendas which should be in alignment but are more often not. Not because both sides don't want the same outcome of better health for you as a patient, but because many may not understand the underlying mechanics involved in arriving at that outcome. Knowledge as we discussed, is empowering. In these pages you will find practical information on the workings of current outpatient primary medical care, and the hurdles that clinic personnel and providers have to overcome to provide care. Developing a better understanding of how the system works may allow you to navigate it with more effectiveness on a personal level and allow more compassion for the individuals working hard behind the scenes on a collective level.

Chapter 4
Scheduling and Appointments

(AKA: Just how long can I wait on hold, and can you please get some better music?)

I often hear comments from the public about their primary care doc *"just seeing as many patients as they can to make money."* I always literally laugh out loud at this statement. I can't speak for every individual physician but I have never personally met anyone who went into primary care for money. There are better and easier ways to support yourself and your family; ones that don't entail huge student loans, ridiculous hours in training that are compensated below the minimum wage per hour, and work requirements that get more demanding the longer you practice, not less. And forget about cost-of-living increases and raises. My friends who went into other fields of work can't believe that our income may go down, not up, the longer that we work for an organization or ourselves. So, not to say that we as a profession in primary care don't make a good living, we do, but not the range that most physicians make that specialize, and not what many patients perceive. In fact, a starting sales job with some companies exceeds the starting salaries for some starting primary care providers, and the starting provider likely has far more student loans. Not that income is an insignificant issue, and we all, not just providers need to feel like the work we do is compensated and valued. But most providers genuinely care about their patients and are invested in doing the best they can. Very few are packing their schedules with as many patients as possible to make as much profit as the day will allow. Most overpacked schedules are simply due to having more patients needing appointments than what is available.

Routine Scheduling

Many of us actually remember when this was done by the usually friendly front desk personnel within each clinic, and there are some clinics here and there that still enjoy this benefit. And if you find or have access to one of these: **celebrate!** It was reassuring to have a familiar face who greeted you by name when you walked in the door. As more and more primary care clinics are run by large healthcare organizations *(In the 2018 Survey of America's Physicians, only 25.7% of primary care physicians identified as a practice owner)* these are becoming increasingly rare. These large entities may own multiple clinics and facilities, and the ongoing trend is to centralize services, including scheduling. This is how it works: when you call for any appointment the person on the phone will answer with your clinic's name, but they are located in an office that may be in a different location and may even be in a different city or state than your clinic. They may have no idea of even where your clinic is, much less the medical assistant or nurse who takes care of you. They can schedule your appointment based on templates for each provider but have no true understanding of how your clinic works. Templates are guidelines that dictate how many patients can be seen in a day and may have certain ratios for wellness/annual exam appointments and routine follow ups and urgent visits. These templates are sometimes controlled by the providers but are increasingly standardized and controlled by systems. This standardization means that all primary care providers employed by an organization within an area or clinic may have to adhere to the same scheduling template. In the past, schedulers within individual clinics knew when a patient called if they might need more time due to complex medical issues, and schedule accordingly or they could ask the clinical staff if this was needed. If a provider and their nurse or assistant control the template they can still determine this. But, if the system has a standardized template this becomes harder to accomplish. So, the patient with 3 pages of medications and medical issues may be scheduled for the same amount of time as the person on one medication and high blood pressure. While there are attempts to determine scheduling based on complexity, we aren't there yet. As a result, appointments are often scheduled incorrectly, or without much thought to what you might need at that appointment. You can see where this creates issues for both you as a patient and the person providing care and creates logjams in the schedule.

When things don't go well in this regard, please don't express your anger at the front desk person. They may know nothing about the fact you needed a note on your Covid vaccine that *"your clinic person I just talked to said to drop by the clinic and pick it up."* Again, you may have been speaking with someone not directly involved with your clinic with no idea of the logistics of your clinic operations. Your anger and frustration may be justified, but it is an ongoing problem not just for you as a patient, but also for the personnel who staff the clinics. Directing your frustration at someone just as caught in the problem as you only compounds the problem.

One scheduler I spoke with told me the worst part of her job was being yelled at or serving as the focus of patient frustrations every single day at work. Most front desk staff will do their best to assist you, but as they are also checking in and taking care of patients with appointments, there may be little time for additional requests. Because of these issues, the workers who are the face of the primary care clinics often don't remain in these positions long, creating even more problems for clinics. If you have a negative experience with scheduling, consider reaching out to the clinic manager or health care organization feedback line to express your concern, as patient feedback is considered vitally important to most organizations. The clinic personnel likely have little to no say in either what caused a problem or how to prevent it.

An even bigger push is to have patients schedule their own appointments online or through an app. Systems like data points because they can be tracked, so they tend to prioritize any change that facilitates data collection to help determine resource allocation. It also costs more to have someone answer the phone than for you to push a button on your phone or computer. If you are tech savvy, online scheduling is a really convenient option, but for many older patients (like my dad), who are a large portion of who interact with the healthcare system, this may not be so easy to use. The unfortunate result of this push is less available personnel to actually staff phone interactions, with ensuing long wait times of unpleasant music and a voice telling you how important your phone call is. If your call were really that important, there would be more people to answer the phone (*and also at the bank, the airline, the DMV…..*).

Types of Appointments

The type of appointment that you are scheduled for is equally important and sets the stage for a successful visit with your provider. Different systems may call them by different names but the general type of appointments are:

Wellness Visits: A routine wellness exam usually entails some review of your history and may or may not also contain a physical examination component. These may also be called "Annual Physicals" or "Annual Exams". These types of appointments have certain requirements from insurance companies and the government that MUST be addressed during those visits in order for the clinic and provider to be reimbursed. The long litany of questions that drive my patients crazy at these appointments are for the most part dictated by outside entities. The staff could probably ask this list in their sleep. The reality is that most clinics participate in programs through Medicare and others that require documenting these questions, history updates, and preventive care services such as mammograms, eye exams, immunizations, colonoscopies and others in the chart. If not documented, clinics may not be paid in full for the care they provide. Entering all of this information can take a sizable portion of the time dedicated to these types of appointments, leaving little time with the provider. As providers we try to use the time that we have left in these wellness exams to focus on areas of the physical exam or symptom review that are important such as screening for age-related conditions that may not come up during routine visits. Do not misunderstand: the questions and history update are important for complex patients of any age, and especially with older patients. It allows for issues such as fall risk, cognitive decline, and social factors impacting health to be evaluated. This is where we can find out that your father is requiring more physical assistance and impacting your mother's health, or that your grandmother is only eating peanut butter and jelly sandwiches every day. These types of concerns often get lost in the shuffle of routine visits, especially when there are multiple chronic conditions, which is unfortunately, many of us these days. This is not usually the place to have a new medical issue or concern addressed. Most providers do their best to evaluate your concern, but do not be offended if you are asked to schedule a separate appointment. While this does result in another charge for you as a patient and more minutes and hours from your day, this request is to make sure that your provider has the space and time to devote appropriate attention to your concern. I have had patients mention what they considered to be a minor new issue at a wellness exam that turned out to be a major health condition, requiring an extensive work-up. While you may be upset at being asked to come back, the resulting time available that uncovers a serious problem is worth your annoyance. You wouldn't want your mechanic to barely glance at your brakes that you mention may not be working well at the end of your scheduled oil and fluid change. It's kind of the same – you don't want to drive off the cliff when you could have prevented it.

Routine: These are general purpose appointments to monitor any type of medical issue which is being worked up or evaluated, and to monitor the status of chronic conditions. These types of appointments are important for patients with chronic issues, such as diabetes or heart disease, to make sure the current plan and medications are adequately addressing your health condition. This is where your provider will determine if your medications need adjustments or if you are due for updated monitoring lab or imaging. The frequency of these appointments is a discussion between you and your provider as some issues need closer monitoring than others. Non urgent, new concerns are also usually addressed at these appointments. While media may encourage you to "make a list" of all of your questions to bring to your appointment, and I have seen individuals literally unroll a 'scroll' of questions. *(In my mind I always see someone dressed in a Medieval outfit blowing a trumpet when this occurred – never failed to lighten up my attitude!)*, the reality is that only some of these can be addressed at each appointment. Not because we do not want to, but again, time and space are required to adequately evaluate issues. Review your questions and decide which are the most important to you to have answered and relegate the others to lower on the list if another appointment is required.

In terms of chronic conditions at routine appointments, it is very helpful to bring any type of health data that you collect at home such as glucose readings or blood pressure measurements. A summary or overview of the data that you have put together, especially if there are pages of it, can facilitate the interpretation. It is also helpful to know what your thoughts are on your data or your medical condition. I have had patients with great blood pressure control whom I found out months into our appointments had always left upset because they thought it should be even lower *(because their friend's blood pressure goal from their provider was lower).* There are often different goals for the same medical condition for different patients, depending on other conditions or factors for you as an individual. Your provider takes into account your personal factors when determining goals for your care. This is especially true when a new study is discussed on the morning news with new recommendations that may or may not apply to you. If you don't understand, please ask. Don't assume that lack of knowledge or concern by your provider underlies what you may have a question about that isn't discussed.

Urgent: These appointments are for new issues, or an unexpected change to a known condition. These can be something as simple as a cold, or as complex as new abdominal pain. Some organizations will only schedule these through a nurse or other person to triage the problem. If you have a deeply concerning new symptom, consider urgent evaluation at an emergency department or at a minimum, please reach out to speak to someone at your clinic or a representative of your clinic. Make sure that you explain your symptoms and not just schedule a routine appointment. <u>DO NOT schedule an appointment such as this online.</u> I have seen patients having new onset chest pain schedule a routine appointment online and later be diagnosed with an active heart attack at the clinic hours later, with more damage due to the delay. If you feel that you truly need to be seen and are running into roadblocks with your usual clinic, urgent care clinics serve as way for any patient to be seen who maybe is not severe enough to need the emergency department but cannot wait until the next available clinic appointment with their primary care provider. Keep in mind that these urgent care clinics may have different insurance coverage than your primary care clinic. It is helpful if you can access an urgent care clinic that is associated with your primary care clinic: your records are available and the urgent care provider has all of your medications and medical history available. At a follow up, your primary care provider can access what was done at the urgent care appointment to determine if additional things are needed. If you have any type of medical concern that you feel could be life threatening, the emergency department is your best option. No one likes to have to go to the emergency department, but if you speak to an on-call physician who recommends this, please follow through. Your worst-case scenario if you go and it was not of major concern is that you spent money unnecessarily. Your worst-case scenario if you don't go and it was of major concern is that you have an event such as a stroke or an infection that has progressed and is now a critical problem or has irreversible consequences.

Telemedicine or telehealth appointments became popular during the Covid pandemic when access to actual clinics was limited. These have been beneficial in a myriad of ways including expanding rural access to providers, facilitating appointments for patients with difficulty getting to a clinic (especially homebound patients), and making appointments easier for patients with time constraints. <u>While a great tool, there are situations in which a telehealth appointment is not optimal or recommended.</u> Rashes may be hard to see on a video, enlarged glands difficult to visualize, lungs can't be listened to. If there is not appropriate support for a clear video it is also difficult to optimally evaluate a patient. Your provider or clinic triage person will use your description of your symptoms to determine whether a telehealth visit is appropriate. Be aware that simply discussing a problem is not equivalent to actually seeing the patient during an appointment. Providers will use data from every source to develop a working diagnosis and treatment plan, including how you clinically appear and interact – so, visual online is not as good as an in-person evaluation for this, <u>and telephone alone is significantly more limiting.</u> There are also state limitations on evaluating patients via telehealth if you are not in the same state as your primary care provider. These were waived during Covid but have been reinstated for many states. If you are in another state and have a significant issue that you know needs to be evaluated, consider going to an urgent care as opposed to waiting for your usual provider to figure out the rules of whatever state you are presently in.

However, this is an ever-changing system so check with your provider to stay updated on this.

New Patient: A special note about new patient appointments. Many patients want their new provider to have every detail of their medical history reviewed. While this may be optimal in the grand scheme of things, it is often not feasible. Providers may receive the equivalent of literally boxes of printed materials and there is no time in an already overloaded schedule to review each and every item in these files. While as a patient you may not know what each test and clinical note means, obtaining and reviewing these can help familiarize you with your own medical history. Often your previous clinic has or will mail (or electronically send) all of your records. If mailed to the clinic you could ask your provider to give you these records after they are reviewed and the significant ones have been added to your clinic chart. Consider keeping these records at home for reference, either summarized digitally or on paper. Also consider putting together a 1-to-2 page health summary that you can keep as well as bring with you to include:

1. Current medical problems

2. Past medical problems

3. Previous surgeries

4. Drug allergies

5. Current medications (include supplements)

6. Recent lab testing

7. Significant procedures such as any heart testing, imaging studies, etc.

8. Known physical findings such as heart murmurs

9. Preventive care reports such as mammograms, eye exams, pap smears

10. Significant social issues that may impact your care

11. How you wish to be addressed: Mr., Mrs., first name, nickname, pronouns etc.

12. Family history of medical issues, especially conditions that have occurred in multiple family members such as heart disease or cancers. Take the time to collect this information from family members.

A caveat to remember during appointments is that as noted above, while your provider is asking you questions, they are evaluating you on multiple levels as soon as they enter the room. They are sorting through mountains of data, based on didactic knowledge and experience, in the background to determine the next question to ask, or the next aspect to evaluate. A patient who looks "good" with a new symptom and a certain set of answers may get one recommendation and routine follow-up. Another patient with the same symptom who looks "worrisome" or has different answers may need urgent imaging or may be sent to the emergency department.

Who Should Be in the Clinic Room?

If you are a cognitively intact patient, this is entirely up to you. Many couples routinely attend their appointments together, while others individually. There is no right or wrong way to this, just personal choice. However, if you have a family member who may have cognitive issues, please consider having someone accompany them. We often have patients with cognitive deficits who are dropped off for their appointments alone. We do our best but often have no real idea of what is occurring at home, if medications are being taken correctly, if the patient is eating, etc. The response from the patient that we often get is "I'm fine" and when asked about any symptom the answer is "No, doing well". It is not uncommon to receive communication from a family member after the appointment asking why something wasn't addressed, or medications refilled, or why we didn't evaluate the rash, etc. The truth is we didn't have the information. The piece of paper that you may have sent never made it to us, or we forgot about the note you sent two days prior. And if you are concerned that the cognition of a family member is becoming impaired, is it important to accompany them and bring this up. Our limited 15 to 20 minute interaction with a patient may not be enough to pick this up. Patients are often fearful of cognitive issues and the limitations it could impose on them, so denial is the norm. The phone call or message expressing concern before the appointment doesn't help us if the patient denies any issues and refuses to answer questions about it. If you bring it up, it sometimes opens the door for us to have a detailed discussion and order testing. Sometimes, patients have another diagnosis such as a mental health problem that is impacting their cognition. I have seen many patients shed tears of relief when they can finally talk about it and learn that it may not be dementia. They relay that they had been dealing with the fear alone, not wanting to worry their family, while the family had been in fear that the patient had dementia as well and didn't want to bring it up to the patient.

Mental illness is another instance in which accompanying a patient could be helpful. If you are concerned about the mental health of a family member, ask them if you can come into the room with them.

Again, some patients will not admit to symptoms when asked, but sometimes will with a family member present expressing concern.

If a patient requires assistance at home, information from the caregiver can be invaluable. Consider being present for a portion of the visit to discuss any concerns about functioning or other issues. Patients who require assistance are as bad as the rest of us at recognizing changes or problems, but the impact can be greater. Unfortunately, the first knowledge that we sometimes have of "weak" spells or worsening mobility is the emergency department report of a fall with a broken hip or head injury.

In my experience many older patients have such fear about being placed into a "facility" or a "home" that they put on the brightest, most cheerful façade they can at appointments. They often deny any issues or concerns. They walk confidently and cover up the fact that their knee hurts and often feels unstable. They don't tell us about the "spells" where they almost pass out. Unless someone accompanies them to let us know that there are concerns, these remain unrecognized by the provider. My own family members have been guilty of this. When asked if they had told their provider about their episodes of a racing heart, they responded *"Yes I did and he said it was fine and not to worry about it."* When I did a little digging, the truth came out that the problem had never been discussed. We all fear losing our health, and it is never easy to face.

Timing

I want to address the often-big elephant in the room of timing and running late or being late. It is such a major source of conflict, and I'm not sure there are any easy answers to this. As primary care physicians we consider your health and needs while you are in the clinic room with us as the immediate priority. When the door closes, short of an emergency, we are yours for the totality of your appointment. If you share that your marriage is falling apart or your best friend died last week, we are going to listen and provide the space and attention that you need to help process that. If you tell us that your spouse has cancer, we will give you time and a safe space to talk about it. If the time runs over your 15- to-20 minute allotment, we don't look at the clock and tell you that your time is up. It goes against our core beliefs and training to not support you. If your elderly parent is in for their routine appointment and requires an extra 5 minutes or more because we cannot get them to quit telling us about their grandchildren in order to focus on answering our questions, we will try to give them that time. We actually really like to be on time and don't choose to run late in our clinics. In fact, it is a MAJOR stress for most providers. We work very hard to achieve adherence to our schedule for both our patients and us, as every minute that we run behind creates loads of stress that we carry through the rest of the day. It means that we often don't get to eat lunch, or that we will have to stay extra late after clinic hours to catch up on administrative work that is piling up. But it is part and parcel of caring for people. Just as your days often don't go as expected, our patient encounters often don't as well. We don't set a timer and walk out of the room when your allotted time is up. Annoyance is easy to reach for but consider gratitude that you were not the one that needed the extra time that day. *(I have personally waited three hours for an appointment before and was indeed grateful my health issue was not the cause.)*

And yes, we may occasionally ask you to reschedule if you are running more than 10-15 minutes late for your appointment. Not often. Not because we don't understand that there may be things outside of your control that caused it, or that we don't care or want to see you. Nor is it because we don't value or respect your time. And also yes, we know that it seems unfair when you arrive on time and we are 10-15 minutes late.

We just occasionally have to draw the line somewhere in order to keep the train on the tracks.

TIPS:

-Understand that the scheduler on the line may know little about your clinic or provider

-Schedule the correct type of appointment

-if possible, formulate a **summary** of your health history and bring with you to a new patient appointment, and have additional records for reference. Keep this summary for future reference.

-Understand that the long list of questions during wellness appointments are required by insurance and government payors.

-Be reasonable with the number of issues that you request your provider address at each appointment

-Evaluate if a family member or friend has an issue that would be helped by accompanying them to an appointment.

-Consider patience when your provider runs late. It could be you next that needs the extra time.

-If your new symptom is truly concerning but you are unsure about the emergency department, always default to speaking to someone from your clinic, or clinical professional to triage you appropriately. Don't forget that urgent care clinics are an option.

Chapter 5
Understanding and Selecting a Provider

(AKA: Where did all the cowboys, I mean primary care providers go?)

I often hear my family members upset because the cardiologist that they go to won't address their shoulder pain, or the gastroenterologist they see for their ulcerative colitis has no response to working up their new tingling and numbness in their feet. These scenarios underlie the reason that you need a primary care provider. These are the professionals who will help you evaluate your new symptoms and determine if a referral to a specialist is needed. The truth is that medicine has become so complex in so many ways that it is difficult to keep up. There are multitudes of medications, therapies and interventions and the list grows longer every year. There is a good chance that if you ask your specialist about an issue that is not considered part of their specialty they may not remember the optimal workup and intervention for it. Just like your primary care provider may not be familiar with the latest and greatest cutting-edge therapy for a condition. Both types of providers have their place and are important, but if you're the owner of your healthcare ship, your primary care provider is your captain. They can help you set a course and bring in whatever crew is needed to get you to your destination.

Optimally every one of us needs and wants a smart, caring, compassionate primary care provider (me included). The unfortunate reality is that care and compassion aren't easily measured on a datasheet and therefore aren't often rewarded in our current system. Every healthcare entity boldly states these qualities as paramount goals in advertising, and likely does want to provide it to their patients. However, they don't know how to effectively measure and compensate for these qualities so it becomes a great slogan with no real support behind it.

Current data shows that there are fewer and fewer primary care physicians for multiple reasons. One issue is there are fewer medical students who select primary care specialties. While medical schools report about 40 percent of graduates enter a primary care residency, that number later turned into just 22 percent, according to a study published in Family Medicine in 2021.[1] There is a projected shortage by 2034 of between 37,800 and 124,000 physicians, according to *The Complexities of Physician Supply and Demand: Projections From 2019 to 2034* (PDF), a report released in 2020 by the Association of American Medical Colleges (AAMC). Of that, between 17,800 and 48,000 are primary care physicians.[2] However, primary care shortage varies significantly by state and is increasing much faster in some states more than others.[3] Much of the public is not aware that many students who complete what is considered a primary care residency, such as internal medicine, choose to specialize. The allure of better compensation, less burdensome paperwork, not having to deal with the complexities of coordination of care and addressing multiple medical issues pushes many toward those specialties. However, it is also important to realize that there is an upcoming shortage across all physician specialties; primary care is just one of the largest areas of current concern. The population of patients needing primary care is becoming larger than the number of providers to care for them. There was a 10% increase in the number of adults 18 and over from 2010 to 2020 according to the US Census, and this percentage is only increasing. Remember that statistic, of only 565,412 primary care providers responsible for almost 80% of the 329.5 million of the US population? These are sobering numbers. Consider that the average student loan upon exiting medical school is now $200,000.00 or more, making lower paying fields such as primary care less attractive. If the average physician can't pay off educational debts within 10 years, their total educational costs will likely exceed $300,000.[4] This is occurring at a time in most physician's lives that they are beginning families and incurring other debts such as mortgages and childcare while trying to pay back these loans. At the other end of the spectrum, the exodus from primary care is equally worrisome. Providers may opt to retire earlier, reduce patient clinic hours or close their clinical practice to move towards more administrative positions. For the providers who remain, burnout is at an all-time high of around 50% in a 2021 survey: worse among women and worse in those in outpatient settings (this means your primary care clinic).[5] Doctors in the U.S. experience symptoms of burnout at almost twice the rate of other workers, citing as contributing factors the long hours, a fear of being sued, and having to deal with growing bureaucracy, like filling out clunky and time-consuming electronic medical records.

Burned-out doctors tend to make more medical errors, and their patients have worse outcomes and are less satisfied, so the emotional health of your provider directly impacts you. No one likes a cranky irritable provider and your provider does not enjoy that state either. A reflection of this struggle is that doctors also have higher rates of suicide than the general population, according to the American Foundation for Suicide Prevention.[6] Additionally, there is data showing that burnout and early exit of providers is occurring with PA's (physician assistants) and NP's (nurse practitioners) as well. As previously mentioned, Covid certainly didn't help the situation, but in many ways just unmasked these problems within our system. In fact, the survey cited above was taken in 2021, after Covid had "settled down" to some degree.

Let's talk for a moment about mid-level providers. These are providers such as advanced practice nurses (nurse practitioners) and physician assistants.

These providers have helped fill the gap in primary care physician shortages and will likely continue to do so. They are a significant reason that we have not felt the shortage so acutely, especially in rural areas. I have had many patients over the years who refuse to see mid-level providers, and I have to admit to many concerns about the quality of care when these types of providers initially entered the scene. What I have determined over the years however is that, just like physicians, there are good ones and bad ones. Although I do think that the many more years of training a physician receives makes a difference, I have found that for typical issues that arise in most primary care practices, mid-level providers are very capable, and are a valuable resource. They often work closely with a particular physician or group of physicians and operate as a team. For difficult cases or any questions, they can access a physician for consultation. Some states allow mid-level providers to operate independently but usually the mid-level has access to physician specialist for consultation through telehealth. Their training does differ from physicians as follows:

> -Doctor of Medicine: (M.D.): requires a college degree, 4 years of medical school and post medical school training called residency *(we often say this is because we live in the hospital during this time!)* that can be from 3 years up to 5 years or more, depending on which area you choose to train in. Examples of residencies are internal medicine, family practice, radiology, general surgery, pediatrics, obstetrics/gynecology, urology and others. Physicians can choose to receive further training, called fellowships, that usually require several more years of clinical work. These include subspecialties such as cardiology, endocrinology cardiovascular surgery, plastic surgery and interventional radiology just to name a few. There are additional even more focused training

opportunities from these areas that require more years of study. An M.D. degree is awarded after completing medical school and requires that a standardized national exam taken in stages be passed. After further training, physicians can elect to take national board examinations in specific specialties or subspecialties. This is referred to as "Board Certified" and requires ongoing evaluation and extra work to maintain.

-Doctor of Osteopathy (D.O.): Very similar to M.D. training but incorporates manual, or hands on, manipulation of joints and tissues to manage patients. These physicians can enter the same type of residency and specialty training as MD's and are otherwise very similar and are considered equivalent.

-Nurse Practitioner (NP): To become an NP requires obtaining a Bachelor of Science in Nursing (BSN), be a registered nurse (RN), complete an NP-focused graduate master's or doctoral nursing program and successfully pass a national NP board certification exam. The different types of NPs are: advanced practice registered nurses (APRNs), certified registered nurse anesthetists (CRNAs), certified nurse-midwives (CNMs) and clinical nurse specialists (CNSs). The NP must select their area of interest (such as pediatrics, primary care, women's health, psychiatry) and receive specialized training in this patient population throughout their education.[7]

-Physician Assistant/Associate (PA): The PA certification is at the level of a master's degree. Acceptance into a program requires a bachelor's degree and successful completion of courses in basic and behavioral sciences as prerequisites. The PA program is 27 months and a certification exam must be passed after completion. As opposed to NP's all students are trained in general medicine and not a particular population. PA's often work with specific specialties after training such as orthopedics, surgery, primary care, etc.[8]

So how to find a primary care provider in the face of a worsening shortage? The reality is that it is difficult and predicted to get worse. More patients have chronic medical conditions occurring at younger ages, meaning that they are accessing the medical system more than would be expected for their age group. In addition, our population is aging and will be skewed toward an older population for the first time in our nation's history. These older patients (of which we will all become if we are fortunate enough to reach an older age) represent the highest utilizers of the health care system.

While many patients can select from a range of primary care providers, some patients may be limited. Some are assigned a primary care provider by their insurance carrier, others may have a very limited list of providers who participate in their insurance, and others may have few providers actually available in their geographical area. In these cases, having access to any provider is a win, and you take what you can get. In areas where there are more providers and options, many providers are closed to new patients. Just because your insurance company lists a provider, it does not mean they are accepting patients. I have had more than a few patients look at a list and decide that I would be their physician only to find out months later, when they needed an urgent evaluation or annual evaluation, that I was not accepting new patients. If your spouse or family member is seeing a provider they are pleased with, consider asking if you can be seen at that clinic. Providers will sometimes work with spouses and families to help facilitate care. You could also look at online reviews but as we all know these venues can sometimes serve as outlets for disgruntled patients (sometimes rightly so) while the satisfied majority may not take the time to report.

An option for some patients is a type of primary care referenced as "concierge medicine" or "direct primary care (DPC). These providers have elected to work either individually or with a formal management organization to provide care. Generally, you will pay a fee per month or year for each which entitles you to general medical care with better access to appointments and better online and phone communication. The difference is that concierge programs are usually pricier and they participate in insurance and government reimbursement programs. DPC programs do not take insurance and your fee covers visits, lab testing and other services, relying completely on fees from patients. The structure varies widely in what is included and offered with each type of practice. The advantage is access is usually better as the provider cares for a smaller panel of patients. The disadvantage is that you are paying additional fees for the concierge model and may have limited items covered by DPC models.

Other types of medical entities to provide primary care are springing up in all geographical areas in an attempt to find better ways for patents to access primary care. There are many models and it may be worth your while to investigate if one of these is a better fit than a traditional medical practice. Remember that regardless of your out-patient primary care, major medical inpatient care is a separate entity.

(A note about moving. In addition to the stress of sorting through your closets and boxing up your world, finding a new provider is an additional worry. I advise patients to research providers in the area where they are moving, seek out and schedule a new patient appointment for when they arrive. Do this BEFORE you actually move in order to not have a break in your care. This is especially important if you are on chronic medications or in need of ongoing monitoring and care. Talk with your existing

provider and make a list of what in the few months after you move will need to be checked or ordered by your new provider. Consider obtaining a health summary from your current provider to take with you to facilitate your new patient appointment once you move. Discuss with your existing provider obtaining enough refills for any current medications to bridge any gaps. Please do not call six months after you have moved requesting an updated prescription refill, and that you are now completely out. We are limited by state laws on prescribing medications and providing care outside the states that we are licensed in.)

Establish Yourself as a Patient

It is imperative that when you identify a provider that you make an appointment to establish care. This allows you to find out if they are open to new patients and introduces you to the provider and clinic. Once you are established patient, it becomes much easier to facilitate referrals, refills, and other related tasks. We will rarely prescribe medications or order tests and referrals for patients that we have not seen. It is not "good care" and for us creates malpractice concerns. For example, if a patient relates that they are on a particular medication but states the wrong name (which happens more often than you might think) and that medication is prescribed, we are liable for any adverse outcomes, both ethical and legal.

TIPS:

-Reach out to your insurance carrier first to see if there are specific providers that you can choose from

-Mid-level providers such as NP's and PA's can serve as additional resources as primary care providers

-Schedule a new patient appointment as soon as you identify a provider to determine if they are open to new patients and to establish care

-Ask if providers that see other family members would consider accepting you as a patient.

-Ask friends and acquaintances for recommendations in your area.

-Consider if non-traditional types of primary care are a better fit for you

-Research and make an appointment with a new provider before your actually move.

References

1.Deutchman M, Macaluso F, Chao J, et al. Contributions of US medical schools to primary care (2003-2014): determining and predicting who really goes into primary care. Fam Med. 2020;52(7):483-490. doi:10.22454/FamMed.2020.785068

2.https://www.aamc.org/media/54681/download, accessed 3/21/23

3. Health Resources and Services Administration. State-level projections of supply and demand for primary care practitioners: 2013-2025. Rockville, MD: US Department of Health and Human Services; 2016.

4. https://educationdata.org/average-medical-school-debt. Accessed 3/8/23.

5. https://www.medscape.com/slideshow/2022-lifestyle-burnout-6014664?icd=login_success_email_match_norm. accessed 3/8/23.

6. https://time.com/5595056/physician-burnout-cost5. Accessed 3/8/23.

7. https:// explore-the-variety-of-career-paths-for-nurse-practitioners www.aanp.org/news-feed/ . accessed 3/8/23.

8. https://www.aapa.org/about/what-is-a-pa/. accessed 3/8/23.

Chapter 6: Medications
(AKA: Why didn't you send my prescription in?)

Our world is becoming increasingly medicated, and as a country we have become a culture of pill poppers. Not a judgement, but a statement of fact. Those of us who are older can remember when the analgesic section of a shelf in the drug store was really small with only aspirin, Tylenol and a few others as options. I actually worked in a pharmacy in a small town throughout high school and college. It was unusual for individuals to purchase large volumes of over the counter (OTC, or medications that do not require a prescription) medications and rare for anyone young to do so.

The number of prescriptions filled per day was manageable by one pharmacist working at a reasonable pace, while also taking the time to assist patients with questions. Prescription medications could be stocked on the front and back of five 3-feet long shelves and some under the counter storage. Not so anymore. The shelves of pharmacies are overflowing with a plethora of prescription medications, and stores are now filled with options for OTC analgesics, cold medications, heartburn remedies, and just about any symptom that you could have.

Let's look at the data: in 2021, the number of prescriptions filled was around 6.4 billion, up from around 4 billion in 2009.[1] In 2015–2016, 45.8% of the U.S. population used one or more prescription drugs in the past 30 days, and 66% of US adults were taking a prescription medication. Prescription drug use increased with age overall, and among both males and females.[2] Additionally, 240 million Americans use (OTC) drugs every year.[3] Nontraditional interventions, including supplements and botanicals, are increasingly popular, and among U.S. adults aged 20 and over, 57.6% used any dietary supplement in the past 30 days, and use was higher among women (63.8%) than men (50.8%). Data also shows that the number of supplements taken increases with age.[4]

These statistics are startling. The business of selling us pills is a huge industry. If we focus on just the prescription side of this, comprising the actual prescribing and filling of medications, it is a time-consuming process for the provider, pharmacy provider and patient. Refill requests are a large part of what clinic staff deal with every day, and because of the sheer volume, many systems have also centralized this process, with hopes of streamlining it. Usually the system works well, but sometimes not. So, what happens when your provider prescribes a medication, or you request a refill?

New prescriptions

New prescriptions are a common area where issues arise.

For example: you see your provider and are told you need additional blood pressure medication. Your provider will have to consider what other medications you are on and how they might interact, what your current pulse and blood pressure are, what your current lab results show (potassium levels, sodium levels, kidney function), what other medical conditions that you have and various other factors. They discuss with you the new recommended medication and they call it in or send it in electronically to your pharmacy and you leave your appointment. If all goes well, the pharmacy receives your prescription, fills it and it is ready when you arrive. You get a mountain of paperwork detailing everything about your prescription and leave the pharmacy. Life is good. But…….as we all know this is not how it happens quite frequently. Let's see where things can go wrong.

-Your prescription is not covered by insurance: You arrive at the pharmacy and find out the cost is around that of a nice weekend trip with your partner. Your immediate thought may be why in the heck did your provider send in something that wasn't covered. In truth your provider probably had no idea of what your insurance covers. Some electronic health record (EHR) [also known as electronic medical record (EMR)] systems may be able to give your provider an idea of what your particular insurance company covers, but often the information is incorrect, incomplete or just not available. What is covered by your insurance has to do with multiple behind the scenes variables that involve "deals" that are made between the pharmacy provider, insurance company and medication manufacturer or distributor. If the pharmacy provider agrees to buy "X" brand name drug from a company, the other drugs the company manufactures can be obtained at a cheaper cost. It is complex and not always logical, and changes frequently. What may be covered one year may not be the next. This is true for both brand name and generic medications. Your provider will usually prescribe what they feel is the most appropriate choice for you as an individual. If not covered, in order to get a replacement medication sent in, the pharmacy now has to contact the provider to find another option. As many systems have centralized prescription requests, this could take hours or longer to access the provider. The same issue can happen again with the new prescription while you wait for this process to unfold. While you wait, your provider is being inundated with phone calls or messages to correct this and becoming as frustrated as you. This is where the patience that I have mentioned so often comes into play. Everyone is working diligently to correct this but it does take time. Anger at your pharmacy or clinic will not speed up the process.

-Your prescription was not sent in: I have lost count of how often I hear this from patients. Do clinics forget to send in new prescriptions: yes. Clinics are busy and things fall through the cracks. But usually on review the prescription shows sent by the clinic and received by the pharmacy in the electronic record, but the pharmacy does not show it was received on their end. I have no good answer for this other than electronic systems have glitches just like your personal devices do. I fervently wish that pharmacies would acknowledge this instead of just telling the patient that their provider didn't send it in, as imparting this information might help avoid anger. Additionally, I have also called in a prescription personally on voicemail to a pharmacy and was with the patient when they went to pick it up and was told that nothing had been called in. When asked to check their voicemail, we were again told that it wasn't called in but was miraculously found when I explained I had personally called it in 30 minutes before. So yes, the ball can be dropped on both sides, but usually it is an electronic communication issue. Calling or emailing the clinic and angrily asking why your prescription was not sent in is only going to make the situation worse and frustrate an already overworked medical assistant or nurse trying to help you. I have actually had a medical assistant sit in my office in tears after being yelled at for the third time in one day due to prescription problems that she had no part in creating and was trying very hard to correct.

REFILL OF MEDICATIONS

This is usually easier and often the pharmacy will fill the prescription if there are remaining approved refills available. If the refills have run out, many pharmacy providers will automatically send a refill request electronically or contact the clinic/provider. If everything goes well, the centralized or local person will "ok" the refill request to the pharmacy and you pick it up the next day. Life is again good. But……things go wrong here as well.

-Processing time: As mentioned earlier, it may take time for your provider or clinic to actually "see" the request if a centralized service is in place. The central service will receive the request initially and based on parameters, either refill the medication or send it to the provider/clinic for further review. If sent to the clinic, the staff will then review and see if based on the provider or clinic criteria it can be filled. This often involves a chart review. If there is a question, the request will then be sent to the provider to review. The provider may then also have to review your chart to determine if the refill can be processed. Lots of steps along the way, and in clinics where they receive your request directly and not through a centralized source, there are also steps that require time, just not as many.

In addition, remember the statistics on how many people take prescription medication? Clinics and systems receive overwhelming numbers of refill requests daily, from patients and pharmacies. This is why most clinics have rules on how long they require to refill your medication. Routine refill requests are important but are considered a lower priority than patients actually in the clinic and communication with patients having urgent issues. Please make reminders for yourself on when your medications run out and send in a refill request at least 1 week prior. It is also easier to have refills updated and completed at your actual clinic appointment. Many providers will approve refill of medications for chronic conditions such as high blood pressure, if appropriate, for up to a year. This avoids most of the previous issues, or at least it gets you off the hook for a year.

Mail order pharmacies are wonderful when they work, and nightmares when they don't. Many insurance plans incentivize you to use mail order pharmacies by rewarding you with cheaper prices. The convenience is nice with the medication delivered to your house on a scheduled basis, and you don't have to stand in line at the pharmacy. The downside is that if things do go wrong, you have to endure the phone tree from Hades to actually get to a live person. That person will most likely hear your issue and transfer you to another, then another. By the time you get to someone who can actually help correct the problem, you have repeated the story so many times that you sound like a robot; a very, very angry robot. By the end of these encounters, you really need that blood pressure medication that is now late in arriving. The really terrible part is that the person that you finally get to that can help, is on the receiving end of all of your frustration. Again, take a deep breath and remember that it is the system that is the problem, not usually the people working in it. They are often as frustrated as you *(although the number of times I have had all the "medical reasons" for something not being filled explained to me by a poorly informed representative on the phone is truly astounding)*. The truth is that if you prefer a local pharmacy, the cost difference may not be that significant, and local pharmacies can dispense a 90-day supply like mail order can. Check with your pharmacy benefits on coverage and weigh the good and bad of both routes and determine which is best for you. Inform your provider or clinic of where you want your prescriptions sent, either mail order or local pharmacy. Whatever is entered into the electronic record is usually set as the default for any ongoing refills of that medication, so make sure you verify that it is being sent where you want, especially if you change pharmacies or use different pharmacies for different medications. The more options you use, the higher the chance that something will be sent to the wrong place.

-Your prescription is not covered: see above. As mentioned, coverage can change and your insurance may no longer provide the medication that you have been taking for years and doing well on. You may have to pay the full amount or be asked to pay a higher co-pay.

-Prior or pre authorizations: As providers we are often asked by patients to contact the pharmacy and explain that they need to continue their current medication or provide coverage for a new medication that isn't on their plan. The pharmacy customer service representatives make this sound so easy when you call as a patient (I know, as I have called to check this process). *"We'll send a form to your doctor and once they fill that out and return it to us, we can process your prescription."* Or you receive this same simplistic information in the mail or electronically. Unfortunately, what you are NOT told is that there are very specific criteria that you must meet in order for them to cover your medication. These criteria are different from one insurance to the next and usually require a significant chart review to answer. They often require a list of every covered medication that has been tried and why it isn't appropriate (side effects that occurred or why it didn't work), if there are mitigating medical conditions that require this other medication, etc. We may not have access to this information if you were on any medication before you became our patient, or if they require information that is not documented in your chart. This results in a phone call from a staff member to you to obtain this information, and the ensuing phone tag. In a day already filled with more than clinic staff can do, these types of time-consuming requests are very hard to accomplish and usually generate a headache for all involved. We do complete these but they require additional time resulting in a longer wait for you. If the request is turned down, there is little more that your provider or clinic can do.

-**Your prescription was not sent in: see above**. In addition, refills are sometimes not filled for other reasons. For example, if you are due for monitoring labs, we may fill your prescription for 30 days and inform you directly or ask the pharmacy to inform you to contact the clinic. If you have not been seen for quite some time your provider may give you a short-term supply and ask you to schedule an appointment. Many patients over the years have expressed anger at these policies, and I have been accused of *"just trying to make more money by making me come in for an appointment."* I wonder if the widespread use of prescriptions (see previous statistics) has dulled our respect for just how dangerous these life-saving medications can be. For example, there are common blood pressure medications that can either lower or increase potassium as side effects. If you have seen other providers and they have added or adjusted medications, interactions with these other medications can enhance these side effects. Or if your kidney function has changed for some reason, these levels could also change. Potassium levels that are too high or too low can literally, stop your heart. So, we would rather you be angry with us than dead due to what was supposed to be a helpful medication.

Contact the Prescribing Provider for Refills

All of our lives are busy these days and we (me included) often take the path of least resistance to get mundane daily things done. This is certainly true with prescription refills. It's easier to contact one main person, your primary care provider, for all of your medication refills. We want you to do so for any medication that we have prescribed, but please DO NOT just send us a message or call us to refill a medication prescribed by another physician, such as a specialist. If another provider is evaluating and managing a condition, they need to take point on managing your refills. We do not know their thought processes on why they chose that medication, nor the parameters of how long they want you to take it, when the dose might need to be adjusted or when the current medication might need to be changed to a different one. We frequently get phone calls from patients who contacted the original prescribing provider's office and were told by staff at that clinic that the provider is out, so call your primary care. **This is when you have to push back.** All providers have back-up providers who are on call for their clinic or specialty who can help you with this. You will have to explain that **they** are responsible for managing the medication that **they** prescribed. If you are in a bind, we may give you a few days of the medication, but please do not be angry at us if we do not agree to just refilling your medication for you. After an appointment in clinic, there may be some of these type medications that we will adjust dosing or agree to take over managing, but NOT without a discussion with you.

Along the same lines, if you see a specialist who gives you a "trial" of a medication and it works, it is not appropriate to be told to "have your primary care provider take over filling this for you" without a discussion between the specialist and primary care provider. This unfortunately occurs on a regular basis with some specialty providers and is a real problem with drugs such as pain medications. We are being asked to take over the responsibility for any adverse effects, long term outcomes, etc. for this new medication that we had no say in selecting. In some cases, we may be in agreement, but again, please do not be angry if we decline. We can discuss our concerns and other options with you at an appointment.

Controlled Medications

The Drug Enforcement Agency (DEA) tightly regulates and controls medications that have the potential to be addictive or abused. These medications are known as controlled substances. The control applies to the way the substance is made, used, handled, stored, and distributed. These substances include opioids, stimulants, depressants, hallucinogens, and anabolic steroids. If a controlled substance has a known medical use, such as morphine, Valium, hydrocodone and Adderall, they are available only by prescription from a licensed medical professional. Other controlled substances, such as heroin, which have no known medical use, are illegal in the United States.

These substances are classified according to Schedules, of which there are 5 categories.

Schedule I is considered the highest potential for abuse with no medical use, such as heroin.

Schedule II includes substances with high potential for abuse, and are dangerous, but can be prescribed, such as oxycodone or Adderall.

Schedule III substances have lower to moderate risk for abuse and include lower doses of codeine and testosterone.

Schedule IV substances are defined as drugs with a lower potential for abuse and low risk of dependence and include drugs such as tramadol and lorazepam.

Schedule V substances are defined as drugs with even lower potential for abuse than Schedule IV and consist of preparations containing limited quantities of certain narcotics, such as Robitussin with codeine cough syrup.

We all know the problem our country is having with opioids. Opioid-involved overdose deaths rose from 21,089 in 2010 to 47,600 in 2017 and remained steady through 2019. This was followed by a significant increase in 2020 with 68,630 reported deaths and again in 2021 with 80,411 reported overdose deaths.[5] Many of these are prescription opioid related, of which we as providers and you as patients share responsibility. I don't know of any patient with opioid abuse disorder (yes there is a diagnosis for this) who awakened one morning and decided *"Hey today I think I'll start my journey to abuse opioids."* They didn't intentionally start down a path that would put them at odds with their provider, create relationship issues and risk their health. They likely had pain that did respond to use of an opioid initially and events transpired from there. It is often a true battle between patients who desire to continue opioids and providers who want their patients to reduce their use or consider other options. It is exhausting for everyone involved and the path of least resistance for many providers is to just refill whatever the patient is on or increase the dose when asked. Which is not always the best course of action in the long run. And keep in mind the findings from a study showing that in 2017, of the approximately 47,600 total opioid deaths, excluding homicides: 90.6% of these were unintentional.[6] When we as providers are reluctant to begin or continue opioids, or try to reduce your dose, it is not because we don't care or lack compassion that you are in pain. It is because we are privy to information now available on what underlies chronic pain, and that opioids are not going to treat this problem well on a long-term basis. We are doing our best based on all the data that we have to provide you with optimal treatment. We want you to be healthy and feel well.

Patients on controlled medications often express frustration on delays with the refills of these drugs. Because of the known risks associated with use of opioids and other controlled drugs, they do require special methods to prescribe, and providers and clinics are scrutinized closely on their controlled substance prescription practices. Many states maintain a database of all controlled medications that a patient has filled. When you call for a refill of a controlled medication, these databases are accessed to confirm that these medications are being taken as directed, and that no other provider is prescribing the same medication. Depending on the medication, you may also have to fill out a controlled substance agreement at an appointment with your provider outlining where you can have the prescription filled, how many you will receive per prescription and how your clinic will provide prescriptions. You may also have to have periodic urine drug testing to confirm that you are taking the medication and not diverting or selling it, and to make sure that you are only taking what has been prescribed. It is also critical that you secure these medications at your home. You or anyone responsible for your care should be the only ones who can access them. We commonly receive calls from patients who have had their controlled medication stolen by visitors or family members. While you may not be abusing or selling these drugs, other people do and will. You are legally accountable for what happens with the medication that you have been prescribed. Secure your medications! You would not want to be responsible for anyone, such as a child, dying from taking your controlled medication (or any medication).

DO NOT share your controlled drugs with anyone. They are prescribed specifically for you. More importantly, it is illegal. Federal and state law prohibits the sharing of prescription drugs that are controlled substances.

DO NOT ask for "early" refills of any controlled medication, but especially pain medications. We are directly responsible for monitoring and making sure that you are using these controlled medications appropriately. If you leave for vacation and forget your controlled medication, you will need to see a local provider where you are currently located for enough to last you until you return. And yes, the reality is that you may be looked at as a "drug seeker" and feel judged when you are seen there. While this feels personal and is truly unfortunate, please understand that you and the provider you see are both caught in the same web. You may be the first of several patients requesting a controlled drug that day that actually has a legitimate request. The truth is that there are patients who use these medications inappropriately, even if you don't. Please recognize how important it is that you accept your part in responsible use and management of these medications.

Most clinics have rules related to how refills are managed for controlled medications. Because of the added steps when refilling these medications, clinics and providers will often have even more strict rules on refills. For example, no refill requests on Fridays, or require 72 hours instead of 48 hours, and no refill requests taken after clinic hours. Most providers will decline to refill controlled medications for other provider's patients when on-call. Providers are scrutinized closely over their use of controlled substances and can have their license suspended for concerns related to their prescribing practices, and whether or not they follow guidelines. I have had patients tell me that they feel as if they are being judged for being on controlled medications and made to feel like "addicts" when asked to "pee in a cup." I reassure them that the questions asked and the rules in place are based on the regulations that we must follow in order to prescribe these medications safely. *Please don't misunderstand our concerns and adherence to regulations as a personal judgment of you.* As providers, we have all been yelled at by angry patients who want controlled medications that we are not willing to provide. No provider wants their patients to be in pain, any more than we personally want to be in pain, or have anxiety, or any other negative symptom. I have sat for hours in meetings with other health care providers reviewing data and brainstorming other effective options to help patients with their pain: we do feel compassion for your symptoms.

The bottom line is that your opinion that you need a specific medication will not push us to risk our license to practice if we don't think a controlled medication is best to manage your condition.

And keep in mind that we also have to deal with the fear of retribution from patients. There are physicians who have been killed by angry patients who were denied these medications. Because of all of the added headaches and fear around their use, many providers have stopped prescribing some or all controlled medications. It is a very difficult path for both patients and providers to navigate. Have a discussion with your provider if you are on, or request to be on a controlled medication. If you cannot agree on how best to treat your condition, consider establishing with another provider. Providers do differ in how they view the appropriate prescribing of controlled substances, although all are subject to the same guidelines and regulations.

If you or a family member are on an opiate, talk to your provider about naloxone (Narcan). This is a medication that can be used to reverse the effect of an opiate in a person who has taken too much or overdosed. This does not just happen in people who misuse opiates but can occur in patients taking them correctly. Higher doses and some underlying health conditions can increase the risk. You can obtain a prescription from your provider but most states will allow you to obtain this from a pharmacy without a prescription. Make sure that you understand how and when to use this medication, as it can literally be lifesaving.

Know your Medications.

While your provider does keep a list of medications in your chart, specialists and others involved in your care may make changes to your medications. These are not always captured by the chart, especially if you see a physician who uses a different electronic health record than your primary care provider. Another scenario is when another provider tells you to take a full tablet instead of your current ½ tablet but forgets to change the dose on the medication list or does change the list but it is overlooked. This can result in dangerous drug interactions, especially if your primary care provider prescribes a new medication based on an incomplete or inaccurate list. Most systems allow you to access your medication list online: use this to review the accuracy of the list. Consider keeping a written list of all of your medications to include prescription, OTC and supplements with you, and make sure that the staff member who checks you in for your appointment updates your medication list in your chart. Don't just say "No" when asked if anything has changed: ask to review the list. This is especially important if you are on multiple medications from multiple providers.

Be consistent with taking medications prescribed. Many patients forget to take daily medication which can lead to lack of an optimal effect. It is often difficult to remember daily medication, especially for a condition such as high blood pressure which is usually not associated with any symptoms. When we don't feel well, we tend to prioritize taking medication in the hopes of feeling better, but when we feel well, it gets lost in the shuffle of a busy day. Try to associate taking the medication with something else that you routinely do during the day such as brushing your teeth or making a cup of coffee in the morning. It is also important to complete a full course of what has been prescribed. Antibiotics are the usual suspects in this problem, and not completing antibiotics is a major issue in creating antibiotic resistance. Also, just because your prescription ran out does not necessarily mean that you completed a course of therapy for a specific condition. I have occasionally had patients come in with uncontrolled high blood pressure who didn't understand that they have to take the medication longer than the initial thirty days in order to keep it controlled. The provider assumes the patient knew and the patient assumed the provider would specifically say if it was needed on an ongoing basis. These scenarios can all be prevented with better communication. If you are unsure and we didn't explain clearly, please ask. When it comes to medications, don't assume.

If you or a family member has cognitive issues, it is imperative that someone assists you or them with this task of managing medication. Daily pill boxes, bubble packed medications and more sophisticated pill dispensers are available to assist patients in appropriately taking medication. There are also services that periodically check on this for patients who need assistance. As mentioned previously, someone accompanying the patient to appointments can greatly facilitate their care.

Generic vs. Brand Name and Why Do Brand Name Drugs Cost So Much:

Patients frequently ask whether brand name medications are better. As a general rule, no. A generic medication contains the same active ingredients as its brand name counterpart, but the inactive ingredients can vary. A generic drug must receive approval from the FDA to ensure that the efficacy of the generic (or how well it does what it is supposed to) is comparable to the original branded drug.

When a new drug is developed it is usually very expensive when it is finally brought to market. This angers many providers and patients. What we don't often speak about however is what it costs a company to develop a new drug. Developing a new prescription medicine is estimated to cost $2.6 billion according to a study by Tufts Center for the Study of Drug Development and published in the Journal of Health Economics.[7] There is a significant timeline of development, research, clinical human trials, FDA review and approval, and post marketing data that a company has to fulfill to actually sell the medication. Only about 12% of drugs that enter clinical trials with humans actually receive FDA approval. The developing company only has a limited period from the time of FDA approval and granting of a patent to recoup the expense of this particular medication, as well as lost capital from failed attempts to bring other drugs to market. So, drug companies will charge large sums to patients to access these medications. Once this patent or period of exclusivity expires, other companies can produce and sell a generic version of an FDA approved medication. As they did not have to pay for the development of the drug, their only expenses are in the manufacturing of the actual pill/capsule/liquid/infusion/etc. once the FDA approves the generic version. Therefore, generic drugs are often dramatically cheaper than the original branded version. Many companies will cease producing the original branded version of the drug once a generic is available.

So, the discussion of how much profit to too much is an ethical discussion that I won't take on. I do take issue with companies that produce a generic version of a medication and charge excessive amounts. They have no skin in the game of development and are not contributing to new medications, they are just looking for profits.

In summary, in most cases generic medications are perfectly appropriate and effective. Some specialists may have specific medications that they prefer you source from a brand name but these represent a small list. Speak with your provider or specialist about this if they do recommend you buy brand name medication. They may have to assist you in getting your insurance company to provide coverage. A final note on prescription medications. As discussed, coverage can vary from insurance payor to payor and from year to year with the same insurance. You can always check into the cash price for a medication and weigh the options of paying cash for the medication you prefer vs. changing to the one your insurance covers. There are resources such as GoodRx, and organizations such as AARP that provide discount options on the cash price of medications, usually generic, to reduce their cost to a more affordable amount. Do your research as you may find many resources that can assist you with cash discounts.

OTC Medications

OTC medications are a valuable resource for patients. Having access to acetaminophen for a fever or headache, or an antihistamine for an allergic reaction is an important tool in managing your health. A major concern is the lack of understanding by many patients that these are true medications and have drug interactions and side effects just like prescription medications. I cringe when I see teenagers for example, taking high doses of ibuprofen on a regular basis, unknowing of possible side effects with ongoing use. The perception is that because it's not prescription, it's perfectly safe. In fact, many of the current OTC medications on the market used to be prescription. The patient information data that applied to these drugs when they were a prescription would scare many away from taking them. It is imperative that your provider knows all of the OTC medications that you take on a regular basis. For example, if you have heart failure, taking ibuprofen type drugs could impact how much fluid you retain and impact your heart failure adversely. If you have active liver disease, you might need to limit how much acetaminophen that you take. Your provider can only advise you on this if they know that you take it.

Supplements and Botanicals

Supplements and botanicals have become a huge market and increasingly used by patients in our country, where they can serve an important role in maintaining health and treating medical conditions. One large national survey reported that 72% of people using herbal remedies were also taking prescription drugs and 84% were taking over-the-counter preparations.[8] What most patients don't realize is that just because they may be "natural" and/or "plant based" does not mean that they are without safety concerns. The supplement and botanical market <u>is not</u> regulated the same as other medications, and there may be more issues with contaminants, potency of the botanicals and reliable sourcing. In addition, like other medications they can have drug interactions and important side effects. This is especially true if you are on drugs for cancer or blood thinners like warfarin (Coumadin). Botanicals can have pharmacological effects similar to prescription medications and can utilize the same drug processing enzymes in your body that prescription medications use. This means that the botanical medication and the prescription medication must compete to use the same pathway in order to be processed by your body. This could result in higher or lower blood levels, impact how well each works or increase side effects of the prescription or the botanical. The unfortunate truth is that most providers receive very little training in traditional medical schools or training programs on supplements and botanicals. Even after an Integrative Medicine Fellowship covering supplement and botanical use, I still encounter ones that patients are taking that I am unfamiliar with. My partners were familiar with only a select few, and this finding is true for most primary care providers. It is a challenge for both patients and providers to navigate this. If you see an oncologist, it is especially important that you discuss any supplement or botanical with them before taking it, as oncology medication interactions are of special concern.

It is important to make sure that your provider is aware of which ones that you are taking and dosages. At a minimum, they can run drug interactions profiles. The limiting factor is that few drug interaction tools contain a comprehensive list of supplements and botanicals to access. So, unfortunately the onus is on the patient to be your own advocate to ensure the supplements and botanicals that you take are safe. There are a few online resources that you can access to help you.

- The Office of Dietary Supplements, a division of the NIH (National Institutes of Health) https://ods.od.nih.gov/

In summary, prescription medications, OTC medications and botanicals/supplements help us to manage chronic health issues, prevent disease, treat symptoms, and overall improve our quality of life. In some cases, they are actually lifesaving. But there is a shadow side. In some ways they allow us as patients to not have to address issues such as lifestyle changes that could impact our health conditions. And keep in mind that medications have side effects, and medication errors can lead to patient deaths. They can be expensive and even when reasonably priced can add up when patients are on multiple medications.

With the time constraints in our current system, they can be a default for providers instead of time-consuming counseling on how to manage a condition. As a provider and a patient, I always review whether the benefit of a medication outweighs the risk. In our current system, you as a patient will need to educate yourself on your medications (both prescription and otc), supplements and botanicals and become *your* best advocate.

TIPS

-Understand your provider may not have access to your unique insurance plan coverage of medications.

-Ask what your clinic policies are on refills and request refills in a timely manner

-Recognize the steps in actually refilling a medication, and the issues that can arise

-Determine whether using a mail order or local pharmacy works better for you, and verify where you want each medication sent

-Contact the provider or clinic who actually prescribed the medication to you for refills

-Understand the regulations around controlled substances and how refills are processed

-Secure all of your medications and do not share them with anyone. They are prescribed specifically for you and could pose a risk to others.

-Know and keep an updated list of what you take, including OTC and supplements/botanicals. Verify this at appointments for accuracy.

-Consider medication reminder aids for any patient with cognitive concerns

-Remember that OTC and supplements/botanicals are medications. Report them to your provider.

-Utilize resources to help you research any supplements or botanicals and how they might interact with your prescription medications.

References

1. https://www.statista.com/statistics/238702/us-total-medical-prescriptions-issued/. Accessed 3/16/23.

2. https://www.cdc.gov/nchs/products/databriefs/db334.htm. Accessed 3/16/23.

3. https://www.fda.gov/news-events/fda-voices/exciting-new-chapter-otc-drug-history-otc-monograph-reform-cares-act. Accessed 3/16/23.

4. https://www.cdc.gov/nchs/data/databriefs/db399-H.pdf. Accessed 3/16/23.

5. https://nida.nih.gov/research-topics/trends-statistics/overdose-death-rates. Accessed 3/17/23.

6. Olfson M, Rossen LM, Wall MM, Houry D, Blanco C. Trends in Intentional and Unintentional Opioid Overdose Deaths in the United States, 2000-2017. *JAMA*. 2019;322(23):2340–2342. doi:10.1001/jama.2019.16566

7. DiMasi JA et al. Journal of Health Economics, Volume 47, May 2016, Pages 20-33.

8. 15. Gardiner P, Kemper KJ, Legedza A, Phillips RS. Factors associated with herb and dietary supplement use by young adults in the United States. *BMC complementary and alternative medicine 739*. 2007

Chapter 7
Specialty Referrals (Consultations)

(AKA: If you don't know, send me to someone who does!)

When something happens to our health, we understandably want to know right away what it is, what to expect and what to do about it. When your primary care provider cannot give you a clear answer to any of these questions, patients usually want to see a specialist – understandably so. When you and your primary provider have been working on a problem and not finding expected answers or results, referral to a specialist is often the next step. It is a double-edged sword, however. Specialists have additional training and expertise in their individual area but may not always have a broader view of your health in mind like your primary provider does. Both are vitally important for optimal care, but understanding their roles will help facilitate your care.

Your primary care provider is usually your go-to provider when you have a new symptom or set of symptoms. They can provide an initial evaluation and determine how to proceed, and if a specialist is needed. They will also manage many of your chronic conditions like diabetes, hypertension, heart failure, mental health concerns. When you and your provider determine that you need a referral to a specialist, there can be situations that arise and create problems.

LONG WAIT TIMES FOR INITIAL APPOINTMENT.

Just as there are shortages of primary care providers, there are shortages in many specialties.[1] As we access the health care system in increasing numbers, this will continue to be a problem. It is not unusual to place a referral to a specialist and be told that the next appointment is in six months or more. Patients are often infuriated when this occurs and will immediately contact their primary provider office for assistance in moving their appointments to a sooner time. Unfortunately, we have no say in this. While we can and often do, call if we consider that you have a problem that shouldn't wait, it is up to the specialist to make the final determination on where you will be put on their schedule. A frustration for both patient, primary provider and specialist. There are just not enough of some specialists to see the volume of patients trying to access them. They are caught in some of the same patient access problems that plague primary care providers.

What can you do as a patient while you wait? Update your primary provider with any changes in your symptoms that would indicate other interventions would be needed while waiting. Ask people you know if they are seeing a specific specialist they like and see if that provider is covered by your insurance. As providers we often develop a network of specialists that we primarily work with and prefer, but we are usually willing to change the referral to a different specialist if you find one that has sooner appointments. I have had patients do this and I benefited by developing a new specialist to work with.

Finally, consider patience: you do not want to be the patient that <u>HAS</u> to be seen urgently by a specialist!

Why don't you and the specialist communicate?

I have heard versions of this more often than I would like. You see a specialist and have testing done and have been put on new medications or have a new diagnosis. You come back in for a follow up appointment with your primary provider who had no idea what has occurred. Patients are often incredulous and then frustrated (as are we sometimes as your provider). Some specialists communicate very well and contact us directly if there is a significant change in our mutual patient's diagnosis or management, and this is optimal. However, others may just send us a copy of their notes. The issue with this approach is that as your primary care provider we may not receive the note, or it may get lost in the sheer volume of notes that we receive every week. Of the hundreds of notes that we receive in a week, most are just updates on routine care. It is extremely difficult to review every single note to find the small percentage of visits that actually contain changes in diagnoses or medications. It is extremely helpful if your specialist drops a quick line to us directly for a "heads-up" that something has changed. But this can be a big ask in a busy clinic day at a specialty clinic.

The above scenarios all imply that the specialist and primary provider share a common EHR. This problem is compounded when they don't. Now the specialist has to mail or send electronically through another portal, a copy of the visit to the primary care provider, who has to review it and manually enter any new pertinent information into your chart. Again, more time-consuming tasks in an already overpacked day. If we read it and don't note it in the chart, reality is we likely won't remember the change by the time you see us again.

To facilitate that we are all on the same page related to your health, make sure that you review and validate or update your medication list online with any changes made by the specialist. Make a note to review any changes with your primary provider at your next appointment. If you keep a health summary, add any new information from the specialist to it.

WHY DO YOU WANT ME TO CALL MY SPECIALIST ABOUT THE CONDITION THEY'RE MANAGING?

This reflects back to the same reasons that we ask that you refill medications prescribed by a specialist, with that specialist. For example, if you are seeing a urologist regularly for recurrent urinary tract infections, the fact that you are seeing a specialist indicates that you have a complicated condition. You have likely taken multiple rounds of different antibiotics, had imaging or additional lab tests or procedures done to evaluate you, or take daily chronic antibiotics to manage the condition. As providers we are concerned about selecting appropriate antibiotics for you because of issues with bacterial resistance. When you call your primary provider and say that you think that you have a urinary tract infection, we may ask you to contact the urologist managing this condition. Not because we just don't want to help you, but because we may not have access to everything the specialist has done or know what the plan is for management of any recurrences. If we place you on an antibiotic and then you find out from your urologist that it was the wrong one and won't work, everyone loses: appropriate treatment is delayed and money is spent on medication that you won't be taking. If you contact the urologist initially, they may manage the problem, or reach out to us directly to coordinate care for you. Having said this, some primary providers are willing to help cross-cover some conditions. It is important that you discuss this with your primary provider so that you are clear about who is managing what.

The same goes for your recurrent lung infections that you see a pulmonologist for, the heart rhythm problem that is managed by your cardiologist, the ulcerative colitis that a gastroenterologist manages, or the rheumatoid arthritis that you see a rheumatologist for. If you have a new problem, then do contact your primary provider first but if it is a recurrence or symptom or flare of an ongoing problem that a specialist manages, consider contacting them directly for management recommendations. If you don't get a response, continue to reach out until you do.

THE SPECIALIST THAT I WANT TO SEE IS "OUT-OF-NETWORK" (NOT COVERED BY CURRENT INSURANCE PLAN)

Patients are often caught in changing insurance coverage. While issues with non-coverage are more prevalent with prescriptions, specialists as well are dropped from insurance coverage networks for various reasons. Similar to medications, your insurance may tell you that all you need to do is get a letter from your primary provider. Again, not that easy and the only success that I personally remember was when a patient lived in an area where there were literally no other specialists in a particular field, and the insurance company approved them seeing someone "out-of-network". We have no clout with your insurance company or their policies, despite how many letters we write, and how logical and straightforward it may seem.

I have had patients see specialists out-of-network to continue care and/or because they had more confidence in a particular specialist. Some insurance plans will pay "some" of the expense of seeing that provider, but your out-of-pocket expenses often do not count toward your deductible for the year.

My specialist said that you can just order the test or medication.

Again, this is not optimal for you as a patient. We only order tests or prescribe medication when we understand and agree with the reasoning behind it. Additionally, ordering and coverage of some testing seems to be accomplished more easily sometimes when initiated by a specialist. Although some specialists will contact us as primary providers to discuss a patient and coordinate with us on ordering testing or medication, it is never appropriate to have that message given to us by a patient. The opportunity for inaccuracies is too high.

As primary care providers, we do try to facilitate any needed testing if your specialist is not geographically close to you and difficult to access. But we do ask that you contact the specialist first to help guide management. It is important that there is direct communication between providers to avoid errors.

Another important piece of data that many patients are unaware of is the time limitation on referrals. They can differ among insurance carriers and can also differ between who you are referring a patient to. For example, your dietitian referral may only allow you 3 months to schedule your first appointment while the one to a neurologist may allow you up to a full year to schedule. If these expire, you must go through the entire process again to obtain an updated referral.

Specialty consultation is an invaluable service for both primary providers and patients when utilized appropriately. Most providers of all fields interact on a regular basis with each other to optimize care for our mutual patients. We are all on the same team with a goal of providing the best care possible for you. However, one important difference in primary care providers and specialty providers is that primary care has more of a focus on illness prevention and optimizing your overall health, while specialists have a specific focus on treating a problem that has already manifested. Unfortunately, our current system seems to place more emphasis on treating illness as opposed to preventing it, and we allot only about 3.5% of our healthcare spending to prevention.[2] Is it any wonder that only approximately 35 percent of all clinicians in the United States, including nurse practitioners and physician assistants, currently provide primary care services; a number that stands in stark contrast to other high-income countries, where the ratio of primary care providers to specialists is generally 70:30.[3]

Remember also that accessing professionals such as dieticians, respiratory therapists, physical therapists, mental health therapists/counselors and other ancillary services often requires a referral. Referrals are easy to place but the difficulty is that insurance plans usually only cover these referrals for certain conditions. To make it even harder, the conditions that are covered may vary from one insurance company to the next. So, if you want to see the dietitian about weight loss, your insurance may not approve the referral at all, while it will if you have diabetes.. If the referral is approved, there are usually limits on how many visits will be paid. Neither the professionals that you see nor your primary care provider have any control over these limitations.

TIPS

-Understand that there is a shortage of many specialty providers. Your primary care provider is unlikely to be able to influence your appointment timing.

-If there is a long wait for specialty appointment, consider asking for recommendations from friends and family on specialists. If you find someone that you would like to see that may have sooner appointments, inform your primary care provider and see if a change in referral is appropriate.

-To enhance effective communication between your specialist and primary care provider, consider asking your specialist to reach out to your primary care provider directly for a "heads-up" if there is a significant change to your management plan. You could also reach out to your primary care provider personally with a quick note to update them on any changes.

-Update your medication list and health summary with any changes made by your specialist.

-Contact the provider who is actively managing a condition with any recurrences or questions about medications or testing related to that problem.

-Avoid requesting referrals or letters to out-of-network providers. Make an appointment to discuss if you feel this is something important to your health.

-Keep in mind the time limitations that are present with referrals and schedule your appointment in a timely manner

References

1. https://www.aamc.org/media/54681/download, accessed 3/21/23

2. (https://healthcostinstitute.org/all-hcci-reports/spending-on-preventive-services-represents-a-small-fraction-of-total-health-care-spending-but-costs-to-individuals-could-be-high-without-aca-protection, accessed 5/11/23)

3. (https://www.healthaffairs.org/do/10.1377/forefront.20181115.750150/full/,accessed 5/11/23).

Chapter 8
Lab Results/Imaging/Procedures
(aka Do I really need this test?!)

No one likes medical testing, even providers when we need it. No one enjoys having blood drawn or testing performed. It's time out of your day, not fun and often costly. But it is a necessary part of managing your health until we develop the cool scanners that you see in science fiction films (hopefully well on the way!). Just a few comments on ordering and scheduling tests.

Urgency of testing.

Your provider should let you know the appropriate time frame in which to have any lab draws or other testing done. It you aren't told, ask. There are some laboratory blood draws which are more urgent in particular clinical situations where your provider has a specific concern, such as glucose levels, potassium levels or kidney function. Routine labs ordered at annual wellness exams, in contrast, are usually at your convenience. Imaging studies are generally considered more urgent as they are used to evaluate conditions such as broken bones, pneumonia, abdominal pain but can also be done less urgently to follow up on some condition such as an unusual finding on a chest x-ray. Make sure that you understand from your provider exactly when they expect you to have the recommended testing done. Most non-urgent testing means that the order is placed but you get to pick the time and place within the time frame you are given.

It is important to understand that some testing is extremely urgent. If your provider orders a study "STAT" or you see this on your discharge instructions, it means that they have a significant concern that whatever you are experiencing could have a serious underlying cause that might need immediate further management such as hospitalization. If you have a test that is scheduled for you by your provider (or staff) the same day, that is usually considered a STAT test and should be done at the time and place that was scheduled for you. I had a patient once that had new leg swelling and I was concerned that she had a DVT (blood clot) in her leg. I had discussed this possible diagnosis with the patient and that I would have my medical assistant (MA) schedule the study for her to be done that day. The MA scheduled the study and informed the patient that the study was STAT and gave her the time and location that day to have it done. The patient left and we noted that the time for her study had come and gone and there were no results. We called her and she informed us that she didn't want to drive to the facility we had scheduled it for and had re-scheduled it for the next day at a location closer to her house. She related that she just didn't understand the urgency that we thought we had imparted, or what STAT meant.

The bottom line is that if your provider has personally worked to obtain a test with a time and date specifically scheduled, there is likely a reason: don't change it without checking with your provider first. If you hear the word STAT, it is urgent.

Remember that timing issue with referrals? The same issues can occur with testing, especially procedures or imaging studies. Many of these have to be approved by the insurance carrier who provides your health coverage before you can actually be scheduled. This is why it can take several days or more for anyone to contact you about a routine ordered test. A significant number of specialized imaging studies such at CT scans or MRI scans will also require a peer-to-peer conversation between your provider and a physician employed by your insurance carrier in order to have the study approved. As you can imagine, the phone tag that can ensue between your provider and theirs can be a nightmare. Once approval is obtained for the ordered study or procedure, there is a restricted time period for coverage of the test. This could be as short as 30 days. If you do not schedule the test within this time frame, your provider and clinic will have to go through the approval process again. For example, my family member was approved for a new pacemaker. As there are activity limitations after and it was non-urgent, they elected to go on a vacation before having this done. When they returned, the procedure was scheduled but when they showed up for the study on Monday morning (having done all the prep work of special bathing, no food that morning, etc.), they were told that the approval for the procedure had expired the week prior. So, the procedure was cancelled and the office had to obtain a new approval and schedule the procedure again. There are so many of these types of details and steps behind the scenes that are required that it is easy to overlook them. While your provider and clinic staff do their best to keep up with these, asking about this at the time you are called to schedule and making a note can help prevent frustrations such as this. The more proactive you are in your health, the more you can avoid these scenarios.

LOCATION OF TESTING.

While most non urgent testing can be done wherever is the most convenient for you as a patient, some insurance plans may pay differently based on the facility. For example, if you have a CT scan done at a hospital, you may pay a higher amount than if you have the same imaging study done at an outpatient radiology facility. Make sure to check with your insurance provider before you schedule to ensure what would be the most cost-effective option for you.

"Cash" prices for some testing, including labs, are offered by many health systems or facilities and may be significantly less expensive. With high deductible insurance plans, some patients are out of pocket for thousands of dollars before their insurance begins to pay. If you are having a major health issue, it may be wiser to involve your insurance so that you meet your deductible sooner. If routine, it may be more affordable to pay the cash price. You will need to evaluate your individual insurance to determine the best approach for you. Cash prices are often cheaper: check with the facility where you are having testing done to see whether they offer this and what the cost is. You will usually be asked to pay at the time of testing with this option. It is key that you ask and pay before the test: if the test is run through insurance and is not covered, you will have to pay the insurance price, which is usually significantly more. For example: your provider orders a Vitamin D level and you have the lab drawn. Your insurance denies coverage for the lab and you receive a bill for $150.00. This same test may only be $50 if paid for at the time of testing and not billed to insurance. Keep in mind however, that paying cash and not using insurance means that any cost you pay will NOT be applied to your individual or family deductible for the year. It can usually be reimbursed through health spending accounts (see section on insurance for details of these accounts). Knowing how much is left on your deductible and when in the year you are having the test done may also help you decide the best approach.

Check with local resources for any discounted testing. Local governments, organizations such as health clubs, hospitals, churches and others may offer programs for discounted wellness labs. Other groups may offer a selection of screening tests, such as screening for carotid artery plaque or abdominal aneurysms for a discounted price. There are some concerns about the accuracy of these screening imaging procedures and some medical groups do not recommend them, while others do. If you choose to have any of this testing done, it is important to recognize that any "positive" findings found on these type tests HAVE to be discussed with your provider. Your provider will NOT receive a copy of this testing unless you provide it. Please do not send or drop off these results and ask for a phone call or e-mail back on the interpretation of the results unless your provider has agreed to this beforehand. When we order tests, we know the reason why and the clinical condition and symptoms (or lack of) surrounding the test, and with this type of situation we do not. You may need to make an appointment to discuss the results in detail.

Preparation for Testing

Another issue that patients encounter is the unfortunate case of showing up for an imaging study, procedure or blood draw and the test cannot be done due to the patient having eaten. This occurs far more frequently than you might suspect. Some tests require fasting and others don't. One type of ultrasound may require that you drink water before and another not to drink water. Make sure that you ask when you call to schedule what the prerequisites are for your individual test. For lab testing, it is common to fast for 10 or more hours (water allowed) before cholesterol or glucose testing. Testosterone levels and some other hormone testing is optimally done in the early morning, thyroid testing may be more accurate if you avoid taking biotin for several days before, and other testing requires that you hold certain medications before.

These are just examples: check with your provider for specific instructions. As primary providers, we may not be aware of the requirements for individual imaging studies or procedures, so make sure to check with the facility where you schedule these for additional guidance.

Scheduling never contacted you for the test.

This is another unfortunate result of the volume of testing done through the health systems. There are many reasons why, such as inaccurate contact numbers in the chart, messages left that were missed, or the order not going through the electronic system to the correct department. This is again why <u>you need to be your best</u>

health advocate: understand what test was ordered and the urgency of it and make sure that your contact information in your chart is correct. If your provider ordered a test, make a note to schedule it yourself, or follow-up with your provider if their office was supposed to schedule for you. Testing ordered through clinics or companies outside of your clinic's EHR is especially vulnerable to being "lost". For example, I left my annual wellness examination with an order for a stool screening test for colon cancer. I saw the medical assistant order the test and the information was in my discharge notes. Weeks went by and I did not receive any communication from the company who would provide the test. I communicated with my provider and the test was ordered again. Again, no communication. After the third time the medical assistant placed the same order, I was contacted by the company. This occurred over approximately 8-10 weeks. If I hadn't been diligent in following up on this, it would have likely been missed until my next annual wellness appointment. The clinic did everything correctly but the system failed. Why? Neither the clinic, nor I, nor the company are sure where the breakdown happened, but it did. The take home point is that you have to be your best health care advocate, as you are the one who will experience the consequences if something falls through the cracks. As this demonstrates, oversights do not discriminate based on who you are. If your provider ordered a test, make sure that you follow up to ensure it occurs.

Screening tests

While most of us are very good about having any testing necessary for a new health problem, it is easy to forget to schedule those tests when we feel well and for which we have no symptoms. These are important and for most patients a necessary part of maintaining their health. These include testing such as mammograms and colonoscopies and are commonly missed by patients, such as what occurred with my colon cancer screening test. Again, please be an advocate for your health and schedule these. If you have concerns about a particular test, schedule an appointment to discuss with your provider. There may be options for testing that you may be more comfortable with. In addition, not every test or vaccination applies to every patient within a certain demographic. There may be individual factors that mean you are not a candidate or do not need a certain test or immunization.

No news is not always good news.

While the volume of results that a provider must evaluate and act on is often overwhelming, you are entitled to a follow up on any test that is ordered. Usually "no news is good news" is true and routine labs with no worrisome findings fall down the priority list of things to address in a busy clinic day. Recognize that abnormal lab values do not always signify a problem, but any significant change in previously stable or normal values should be addressed. Again, ask your provider before you leave when you should expect communication on your results. Providers know generally how long it may take to get results back, but in a busy day of seeing multiple patients they may forget to relay this to you. Also be aware that clinics and providers differ in their policies on this, so ask before you leave your appointment. If you have not received any communication within the timeframe discussed, then reach out. If you do not receive a response, continue to reach out until you do. The key is having an agreement with your provider on expectations for follow-up. This can prevent frustration on both sides and unnecessary e-mails and phone calls. More on this in the next chapter.

TIPS

-Make sure that you understand and confirm with your provider when the testing should be done.

-STAT testing (always) and testing ordered by your provider for a specific time (usually) are considered urgent.

-If a test is ordered and you have not been contacted, first reach out to the facility where you were told to schedule, and then to your provider's office if urgent or the facility does not have the order for the testing.

-Inquire as to what the approval period is for a scheduled procedure or test (not usually laboratory blood testing), and schedule within that time frame.

-Check with your insurance on where the most cost-effective location/facility to have your testing done. Sometimes cash prices are more affordable than filing it with your insurance.

-Check with local resources for any that offer discounted testing.

-Ask if you should fast or if there are other recommendations necessary for a specific test.

-Check with your provider and make sure that you are aware of screening recommendations for testing.

-Confirm that the contact information in your chart is correct.

Chapter 9
Testing Results

(AKA: I saw my results! Am I dying?!)

Timing of results.

We are curious creatures, especially about ourselves. If there is new information about us, we usually want to know it right away. In a perfect world, after you have testing done, your provider would evaluate the results first and the clinic would contact you with the interpretation of those results. The unfortunate reality is that we live in a world of instant information gratification. To appease this, health systems release all results, as soon as they are available, to patients. This can be suboptimal in that patients often see results before we as providers have time to see them, leading to panicked phone calls, often unnecessary anxiety, and worse: a new diagnosis read on a screen, as opposed to hearing it from your provider. They are your results and you have the right to view them. However, interpretation should optimally come from the provider that ordered the test. It is true that there have been results that were missed leading to adverse outcomes, and legislation has been passed to ensure patients can see their results because of this. I am not implying that patients should not have access to results. But I have seen far more issues with patients viewing abnormal results in a setting with no one to discuss these results with and/or help, interpret and plan, than issues from missed results.

For example, consider a scenario of a pregnant patient, who just had an ultrasound for concerns about her baby not moving as much. She leaves the ultrasound facility and while enroute to her house receives the e-mail that her results are available for review. She looks at her account and the ultrasound results, reading that her baby has died. She now has to continue driving or pull to the side of the road to integrate this information alone. While there is no good way to receive this kind of news, I offer that this patient would have been better served to receive a personal call from her provider, whom she has a relationship with, to discuss, offer emotional support and guide her through the next steps. I have personally received panicked calls from patients who learned about their breast cancer, lymphoma and other cancers by reading it on a screen while at home alone or at work. Equally troubling is when a patient reads that they have a new "mass", "nodule", or "tumor" on an imaging study and the patient immediately interprets this to mean cancer. The results may say something along the lines of "Differential includes *'insert whatever type of cancer here'*" in the list of possible things the finding could represent. Many of these findings represent benign conditions and not cancer, but the radiology physician who read the image has included it as a possibility. The patient may need serial monitoring or no additional follow-up at all. Patients must endure the same level of unnecessary anxiety as the patient who actually does have cancer, until the results can be discussed.

I submit that providers should have an opportunity to review results and personally contact their patients before the results are released. A short interval could optimize how the results are delivered and provide often much needed support, along with answering questions and providing guidance. Consider giving your provider time to review your results and contact you with recommendations first.

INTERPRETATION OF LAB RESULTS.

As primary care providers we receive a tremendous number of communications from patients on a daily basis. It is often difficult to sort out the urgent or problematic issues that need an immediate response from the routine questions. One of the items that often fills up "in-baskets" are questions about routine lab results. When there is often a "button" to ask your provider a question at the bottom of the screen where you view your lab results, it seems natural to do so. I would ask you to consider whether the question is really necessary at that moment, or could you allow your provider time to review and respond. Keep in mind that it took years of training to interpret the results in the context of your individual health. "Dr. Google" has all the lists of possible things that an "elevated BUN" can mean for example, none of which may be applicable to you. I have received literally hundreds of calls over the years on this by concerned patients that there is something wrong with their kidneys, while the cause is often that the patient fasted for their labs.

Normal is subjective and in life we know this varies depending on the group you're in or your culture. However, we expect that "normal" in healthcare is a more concrete concept. The reality is it is not exactly concrete. "Normal" lab results are determined by population studies and are based on the range of where 95% of apparently "normal" individuals' results would fall. There is 2.5% of this "normal" population who had results higher than this range and 2.5% who had results lower than this range, but their results were normal for them. This is just a statistical derivation. So, your lab value that is slightly higher or lower than the "normal range" listed on the lab results may actually be your normal. Remember that <u>normality is relative</u>. The interpretation of any abnormal result is based on your individual factors. If there is a slight abnormality, your provider may ask you to repeat that lab to determine if any additional testing may be needed. Additionally, there are times when a result in a normal range is actually abnormal: if your calcium is elevated, but the hormone level that controls calcium levels is in a "normal" range, this is actually abnormal. So, the concept of "normal" is not as straightforward as looking at a range on the results page.

Lab values can also fluctuate due to many factors within an individual patient from day to day. So, even your lab values can vary, and that is why you may be perfectly healthy and see a result that says it is outside of a normal range. Your provider can interpret whether this is of concern or not. We often say that these are within an acceptable range rather than just "normal".

There are also labs that we use to monitor a particular condition. Abnormal lab results, even when significant, do not always need intervention. If the lab result is abnormal but is stable, no additional intervention may be needed. For example, if you have chronic kidney disease, the lab tests that reflect your kidney function may always be outside of the "normal range". In this case, we are more concerned with any changes in that stable abnormal value. And while some changes are important and need intervention, other changes may not be significant, meaning that no intervention is needed.

Most labs do have "critical" values that will trigger a technician at the lab to reach out immediately to a provider or clinic to inform them of the lab value to address. This covers most issues that could be life threatening such as potassium levels that are significantly out of range.

Having said the above, if you see a result that is dramatically out of the normal range and you do not hear from your provider, please reach out. For example, if you have diabetes and your glucose is 400 and you do not receive a phone call from your provider (I confess this has happened to one of my patients), definitely call and be loud about it. My patient did and we immediately addressed it, and this prompted process changes within my own clinic.

IMAGING

Imaging studies are a bit of a different animal. Urgent or STAT studies require immediate follow-up and your provider should contact you with these results and recommendations as soon as the results are available. Non-urgent studies share some commonality with lab results in that routine results may require a few days for your provider to contact you. Keep in mind that there are often findings on imaging studies which are incidental and have nothing to do with why the study was done. Sometimes these are important and sometimes they are just findings that will not impact your health. Because of this, please reserve judgement on any imaging result until you receive feedback from the ordering provider. A mass on a lung CT scan (CAT scan), for example, could represent cancer, or could represent a benign growth that will never be an issue for you. If there is a concern, please make sure that you complete any additional testing ordered. This is profoundly important, and where you have to be your best advocate. If your provider tells you that you need a follow-up CT scan of your lungs in 6 months, make a note and prioritize this! While there are some mechanisms to help remind you within the EHR systems it is imperative that you do not rely on this. It is your health and you will have to deal with the outcome if the system fails. Determining who is at fault at that point does not reverse any negative outcomes. So, make sure that you prioritize any recommended follow-up testing. Also, please contact the provider that actually ordered the study to discuss results. Many patients reach out to us as their primary care providers to inquire about their results when a specialist has ordered the test. Similar to medications and medical problems, we may not have all the information on why a particular test was ordered, so the interpretation of a test is more challenging.

Procedures

Usually, the results of a true procedure, such as a colonoscopy (evaluation of your colon with a scope), are discussed by the specialist doing the procedure. Make sure that you have a follow-up appointment with your specialist or your primary care provider if the test is abnormal.

Prioritizing

When waiting on or reviewing results, consider whether a phone call or an e-mail with your provider is necessary. Is it curiosity or does it constitute a true concern, such as clarifying a medication recommendation or providing information that could impact interpretation? Are there multiple questions that would be better answered at an actual appointment? I suggest this review of the underlying reason because of the overwhelming volume of communication that most clinics have to deal with in our current system. Remember that each individual communication has to be opened and read in order to understand the urgency of it. This means that the more urgent communications may have a delay in being addressed as the clinic staff has to wade through all the communications to find them and prioritize them. Consider taking a short pause to evaluate your concern and act accordingly.

TIPS

-Confirm with your provider before you leave your appointment, or before you end any communication from the clinic, when you can expect to hear from them on the results of an ordered test. Understand your clinic's policy on this.

-Understand that abnormal values on lab results or findings on imaging studies may or may not be of any clinical concern.

-Try to limit communication to your provider about results that are slightly out of range on routine lab results and allow the clinic to contact you.

-Do contact your provider if you see a lab test that is dramatically out of range and you have not been contacted.

Chapter 10
Paperwork

(AKA: The bane of everyone's existence)

When electronic records became an integral part of clinical care, one of my greatest hopes was that the amount of paperwork would be reduced. This, along with other hopes and dreams related to electronic records I have released into the place where dreams go to die. What it feels like is that we have a similar amount of paperwork to fill out, AND the ever-increasing demands of the electronic medical record.

Patients often drop off paperwork at the front desk to be filled out. While some of these forms, applications, etc. are not time intensive or complicated, many of them are. They require a detailed review of your medical records to find the specific information required. In addition, some of them require an opinion on how fit you are for a specific activity or living situation, as an example. These issues are best discussed at an appointment to go over the details of what needs to be filled out, and to address any specific questions or evaluations that are needed. Please do not take offense if after we review the paperwork we ask you to schedule that appointment. To prepare, please bring with you pertinent summarized information such as a timeline of events and any records if you are asking for medical leave from work, or results of outside testing for a release for some type of activity. This ensures that the correct and pertinent information is included on the forms.

Chapter 11
Electronic Health Records (EHR or EMR)

(AKA: This was supposed to make things easier- what the hell happened?)

Electronic medical records were heralded and should have been the answer to streamlining the care of patients and allowing providers to spend more time with their patients (and not having to read provider's illegible scribbles!). Now we can do away with multiple volumes of 5-inch charts on a complex patient. No more digging through page after page to find the results of that one heart test from 2 years ago. But. There's the big BUT. Some of the streamlining and ease of accessing information did happen, BUT it came at a high cost to both providers and patients.

Providers

While we can access records more easily, track and graph lab results and blood pressure, we now have a computer in the room that often requires more attention than our patients. Instead of evaluating our patient as we talk with them and taking in all that non-verbal information, we divide our attention between our patient and the screen: make eye contact, enter data, look up again, enter more data, eye contact, look up a result, do an exam, back to the computer. It's as if the computer has become the most important entity of the encounter.

Systems have tried to address this problem by hiring personnel who are also in the room and enter information into the computer during the entire encounter, but the provider will still have to address and correct and expand on the notes after. Some providers as an alternative, utilize medical assistants to enter data and place some orders in the room. These interventions do allow the provider to interact more with the patient but are expensive and usually not supported. I personally elected to review my patients charts before the encounter and only open the computer if necessary. I, and my patients were much happier. The patients felt like they actually had my full attention, and I felt less distracted. But the cost of this was more time after appointments playing catch up. Unfortunately, the EHR dominates not only the encounter, but a majority of our clinic hours now. I call it *"feeding the beast,"* and it is a beast. It requires constant time and attention and is always hungry for more data and input. It will eat you alive if you aren't on your toes. The amount of data entry required is enormous and many providers have honestly entered meaningless data on patient encounters by just clicking on data points or reloading previous data because of the demands of so much data entry. As a result, many of our notes are not helpful, but instead full of information to fill the page and check the boxes for the medical systems and insurance providers, in order to be reimbursed.

Trash in = trash out.

So now instead of digging through mountains of paper, we dig through mountains of digital data to find the "pearl" that will help us manage our patients.

Outside of patient encounters is the dreaded "inbox" or "taskbox" or "inbasket." This demon goes by many names. It is where every test result, prescription refill request, paperwork request, patient phone call, patient e-mail, outside record, note from specialists, communication from the system or other providers drops in. As soon as you address one thing, two more drop in. It is one of the most frustrating issues in primary care and a significant contributor to burnout. Keep in mind that most of these items require time and focus to appropriately address. We know that sometimes patients' lives are at stake, and we cannot afford a lack of diligence. Maintaining such a high level of focus at all times during patient interactions and addressing these items is exhausting. In order to just physically leave the clinic, many providers work on these "inbaskets" after hours at home (after dinner and putting the kids to bed) and on weekends (in and around sporting events), cutting into the little free time available. It's like having a bag that you drag around and every second of every day it is filling up. Mondays and returning from any actual time off are days dreaded by every provider that I know and many dedicate a day off to just play catch up.

Artificial Intelligence (AI) provided some hope for improving the efficiency of generating usable notes. But as with current iterations of notes, there is much redundancy and it is difficult to find the important information amongst all of the "filler" data. Maybe this will evolve into a useful tool as AI becomes more advanced, but at the current time it has not offered much in the way of improvement.

The more upstream issues that EHR has created are reducing patients, patient encounters, and providers to data that can be collected and put on a spreadsheet to evaluate. The problem with this approach is that we as patients and providers are more complex entities than can be assessed by simple digital data. The optimal care of patients is multifaceted and any attempts to allocate resources based simply on data points without understanding the front-line issues at the level of care provision will fail. I found it fascinating that the personnel managing health care systems in general fail to see the impact of what is implemented in one area has effects in other areas. It's like a spider web: if you pull on one silken thread, the whole web is impacted and moves. I cannot see this improving as we continue to move the policy makers in systems further away from the actual clinical side of care. I suspect that everyone is diligently managing their individual areas but just don't have enough of the big picture. As I was writing this section, an acquaintance in an MBA program had a person in their class on business management systems comment on his direct experience with a large health care system he spent some time in meetings with. He related that he listened to a lot of discussion from one area of management on the difficulty of retaining staff in the system, and of how many were leaving for better compensation. There was a lot of brainstorming on ways to retain staff. Then, the immediate discussion after was on how excited they were to have the new $50 million dollar building go up (and funded by the system itself, not outside funding). He asked why they didn't put off the new building and use those funds to pay and retain staff and was met with bewilderment. I mean, who wouldn't want the latest and greatest facilities, even if not fully staffed?

As this encounter demonstrates, his suggestion just does not align with our current model of a successful business – business entities should always be growing and expanding to compete. The focus is on growth as a measure of success, whether that is new patients, new buildings, new markets or new technology to offer. There is not a primary focus of taking care of your current system, which is true for business in general, and not just healthcare. I find this interesting to consider, for example do you know in medicine what we call ongoing unchecked unregulated growth in the body? Wait for it………..**Cancer.**

It continues to grow despite expending and damaging the health of the very thing sustaining it.

Personnel

Clinic staff including schedulers, medical assistants and others also struggle with many of the same issues. I have heard medical assistants express feelings of being burnt out as well due to hours sitting at a computer. They also express that the reason they entered their fields was to interact and support patients, not sit at the computer entering data. This issue cuts across all levels.

Patients

From a patient perspective, I have also sat in the chair in an examination room while my provider looked down for much of the encounter at a computer. I have also been in one where someone entered data while the provider interacted with me, and in one where the provider was alone and didn't engage the computer. I can say definitively that not having the computer open was the best and having someone enter the data a close second (and maybe more efficient). As patients it is difficult to have any real impact on this. Maybe relaying to the health care systems your preference could impact.

Data on these issues

To add some data to the impossibility of maintaining our current system in primary care, in a study headed by Dr. Justin Porter, M.D., at the University of Chicago School of Medicine and published in the *Journal of General Internal Medicine,* researchers found that in order to provide guideline-recommended care, a primary care physician would require nearly 26.7 hours per day.[1] *That might be a real problem in a 24-hour day.........*

Porter comments on discussing patient views: *"If you do surveys with patients about what frustrates them about their medical care, you'll frequently hear, 'My doctor doesn't spend time with me' or 'My doctor doesn't follow up [...] I think a lot of times this is interpreted as a lack of empathy, or a lack of willingness to care for a patient. But the reality—for the majority of doctors—is simply a lack of time."*

The 2021 survey of physician burnout revealed that bureaucratic tasks, as opposed to caring for COVID patients, topped the list as causes, aligning perfectly with the study by Porter.

Comments from this survey:

"I barely spend enough time with most patients, just running from one to the next, and then after work, I

spend hours documenting, charting, dealing with reports. I feel like an overpaid clerk."

And

· *"Where's the relationship with patients that used to make this worthwhile? Everyone is in a foul mood."*[5]

It is overwhelming: in one clinic of 7-8 providers, approximately 18,000 to 20,000 pieces of information/communication have to be handled monthly! As these numbers have increased and continue to increase, the staff needed to adequately support it has not. The increased demands of addressing all of those pieces of information mean that workdays can be more intense with productivity demands that can seem unattainable. Gone are the days of discussing patient care with your colleagues in order to obtain another opinion. Gone are the days of sitting down for lunch… not in front of your computer. This is not just a reminiscence about the good ole days. In terms of mental health and stress management, these demands do not combine well with the fact that the US does a poor job of creating an environment conducive to work-life balance.

According to one review in 2022, the United States is the country with the joint fewest days of (statutory) paid leave (0) and the second lowest number of paid vacation days in the world (10).[2]

Some health care systems do grant paid time off (PTO), but in most instances any time a clinic is closed for a holiday or an employee is sick they are required to use their paid time off. And let's not forget that all of this sitting in front of a computer by clinic providers and staff is a change to a more sedentary lifestyle. Many of these clinic employees spend the majority of their week at work sitting in front of a computer.

Research has linked sitting for long periods of time with a number of health concerns. They include obesity and a cluster of conditions — increased blood pressure, high blood sugar, excess body fat around the waist and unhealthy cholesterol levels — that make up metabolic syndrome.[3]

Electronic health records are here to stay. In all fairness they have improved some aspects of patient management. It just became too easy to use the data that is generated to develop policies without giving thought to the consequences. Which is a widespread problem in our current culture. There are significant issues in primary care with EHR that will need to be addressed going forward. While I do think this can be improved, it will require a team approach of both administrators and the personnel actually providing clinical care to solve. It is imperative that front line workers be involved in these decisions for them to be effective on all levels, not just on a spreadsheet. While you cannot fix this as a patient, you can have a discussion with your provider to clarify expectations on your care and ensure that you and your provider are on the same page. Hopefully, this information gives you better insight into why your provider and clinic staff may be distracted, and why it may take a frustrating number of days to receive a response to your question.

TIPS

-Extend patience and compassion for the clinic personnel as they navigate the electronic health records. It is overwhelming.

-Evaluate the urgency of your requests and allow enough time for these to be completed by the clinic personnel

References

1. Porter J, Boyd C, Skandari MR, Laiteerapong N. Revisiting the Time Needed to Provide Adult Primary Care. J Gen Intern Med. 2023 Jan;38(1):147-155. doi: 10.1007/s11606-022-07707-x. Epub 2022 Jul 1. PMID: 35776372; PMCID: PMC9848034.

2. *(https://resume.io/blog/which-country-gets-the-most-paid-vacation-days, accessed 5/10/23)*

3. *(https://www.mayoclinic.org/healthy-lifestyle/adult-health/expert-answers/sitting/faq-20058005)*

Chapter 12
Provider "Grading"

(AKA: There is no studying for this test!)

As providers we are increasingly being mandated by systems to reduce costs, improve patient experiences and improve quality. These are worthy goals, but the problem is the measures by which systems evaluate these. It is difficult to measure care and compassion, and what a patient perceives as "quality." Systems use patient ratings and reviews to help evaluate, but one difficulty is that the individual patient perception of what care, compassion and quality care entail differs. Also, systems use "quality of care" measures in addition to patient reviews, to evaluate an individual provider or group of providers' performance. Some of these measures are inherently flawed, and the patient experience reviews may reflect issues that a provider or clinic have no control over. The unfortunate reality is that many systems, including government systems, use these flawed measures to help determine payment to providers and clinics.

Patient Reviews

Most of us at some point have used an online review to decide which hotel to book, which company to use, and yes, which provider to choose. There is data showing that reviewers are more likely to talk about negative experiences, because of a heightened emotional response and are more likely to do so unprompted.[1]

Some systems will reach out to most patients after their encounters to obtain data to address this. But again, busy patients may not be open to the time to reply unless they had a stellar or subpar experience. As discussed, the patent-provider relationship is complex, and there are multiple negative issues that pressure it. For example, a patient presents with a cold. The provider determines that the cause of the patient's condition is viral and provides recommendations on management. The patient requests antibiotics and because the underlying cause of the cold is thought to be viral, the provider declines to prescribe them. Usually this can be resolved with education and discussion. But occasionally a patient is adamant about needing the antibiotics based on previous experience and the visit ends in a negative manner. The provider was following guidelines in what they considered the best care for the patient. But the patient leaves and provides a scathing review of the quality, lack of care, etc. by the provider. A patient with multiple complex medical problems who had waited two months for an upcoming appointment sees the review and cancels and has to now wait another two-three months to establish with another provider. So, a negative review of a provider or clinic can lead to a patient "doctor shopping" resulting in fragmented care based on incomplete or non-factual information.

Fragmented care can then be associated with higher health costs, completely undermining the initial intent of the measure. Physician rating websites have utility but are imperfect proxies for competence [2,3] While a provider who is a problem and provides poor care should definitely be "outed" so that other patients aren't subjected to the same, reviews can be personal and vengeful and not related to quality of care. I had a patient in the past who provided a long diatribe on how terribly they were treated and harassed by the staff after their appointment. They provided so much detailed information that it was easy to identify who the patient was. The only problem was that much of the information about the clinic was a complete fabrication and the harassment by the staff was an attempt to help facilitate a referral that the patient had agreed to at the time of the appointment. When I asked that this review not be published *(the only one that I had ever requested this of)* I was told that regardless of what occurred, this was the patient's experience and for them it was the truth. That is when I personally elected to quit reading most individual reviews. While most were positive and contained helpful information, human nature is such that I, like most, tend to focus on the negative, not the positive. They only served to increase my frustration and burnout. These reviews can also be related to issues that the provider has no control over such as how the patient interaction portal works. Patients are encouraged to provide feedback on their experience and may have no idea that these may be tied to compensation in some way. A patient trying to be helpful providing information and a poor review due to the parking outside or the temperature being too hot or too cold most likely doesn't know that their provider could be held personally accountable on some level for these issues. The frustrating issue is that as a provider if compensation is partially tied to these reviews, it can be difficult to accept. Whether you are following guidelines and your patient disagrees, or there are issues that we have no control over. As opposed to encouraging us to personally conduct an honest review of how we provide care *(never an easy task as humans to accept our deficiencies in the best circumstances)*, it ignites anger at the injustice of the system. Most of us would welcome feedback on our patient experiences and the chance to improve service if they were not tied to our performance review.

QUALITY METRICS

As mentioned, an additional way that primary providers (and clinics) are evaluated and this information used as a basis for compensation is by what are termed quality metrics. These are based on straight forward data collection such as what percentage of your patients with diabetes had an HBA1C (a test that is used to track how well the blood sugar of a patient with diabetes is controlled) within a given amount of time, or what percentage of your patients had recommended screening tests such as colonoscopies or recommended vaccinations such as pneumococcal (a type of vaccine to help prevent a certain type of pneumonia). Many of these are recommended by the government if you participate in a program such as Medicare. This seems reasonable on paper, but again the clinical aspect of this is missing. As providers we can order lab testing but have no control over whether a patient chooses to have it done. We can order a colonoscopy, or mammogram; recommend a vaccination or pap smear, but a patient can decline.

If you do not want to have a recommended test, just let your provider know so that this can be documented in the chart, although don't be offended if you continue to be asked at future visits. We do not want to assume that you have not changed your mind. In addition, some data, such as did a patient with diabetes have an eye exam, or did a woman have a pap smear, can be more difficult to capture by a computer system. If your gynecologist or eye doctor does not share an EHR with your primary provider's office, this data must be collected from the outside provider and then manually entered into the system. A large ask of an already overburdened staff. These measures or metrics can be helpful but systems need to understand the role that standardized quality assessment tools can have on care practice, reflecting the need to be thoughtful when constructing such measures.[4] Holding providers accountable for issues outside of their control is discouraging and frustrating.

On the flip side: if you know that you are due for a recommended test based on guidelines, please inform your provider. We can absolutely miss things and appreciate any reminders!

TIPS

-Be mindful of the information that you provide on patient feedback. Be honest and thoughtful with commentary.

-Realize that your reviews may impact the reimbursement or compensation of your provider or clinic. If there is a significant problem reach out to a clinic manager or patient representative directly.

-If your provider recommends or orders a test, please make sure that they know if you decline, so this can be documented. Otherwise, please make time to have these completed. Your provider or clinic can be held accountable if you do not.

References

1. *(http://cdn.zendesk.com/resources/whitepapers/Zendesk_WP_Customer_Service_and_Business_Results.pdf accessed May 9, 2023)*

2. Murphy GP, Awad MA, Osterberg EC, Gaither TW, Chumnarnsongkhroh T, Washington SL, Breyer BN. Web-based physician ratings for California physicians on probation. J Med Internet Res. 2017 Aug 22;19(8): e254. doi: 10.2196/jmir.7488. http://www.jmir.org/2017/8/e254/ [PMC free article] [PubMed] [CrossRef] [Google Scholar]

3. Okike K, Peter-Bibb TK, Xie KC, Okike ON. Association between physician online rating and quality

of care. J Med Internet Res. 2016 Dec 13;18(12): e324. doi: 10.2196/jmir.6612.

http://www.jmir.org/2016/12/e324/ [PMC free article] [PubMed] [CrossRef] [Google Scholar]

4. Goitein L, James B. Standardized best practices and individual craft-based medicine: a conversation about quality. JAMA Intern Med. 2016 Jun 01;176(6):835–8. doi: 10.1001/jamainternmed.2016.1641.

http://jamanetwork.com/journals/jamainternalmedicine/article-abstract/2521828. [PubMed] [CrossRef] [Google Scholar]

CHAPTER 13
INSURANCE

(AKA: Do I need a college degree to interpret this? Or... I have a college degree and still don't understand this!)

Anyone who has health insurance likely understands how complex it can be to navigate. You think you are following the dictates of your policy then you get a huge bill in the mail for non-covered charges. It is also frustrating for clinics and providers; you think you are following the dictates of the insurance carrier and then the test you ordered for your patient is denied. And patients are usually extremely upset by this – as are we as your provider. The reality is that even within the same insurance carrier there may be a multitude of different types of policies, and each may cover different things. It is always a good idea to print out and have on hand for reference what your insurance covers or "allows" and does not in terms of procedures, well visits, urgent visits, emergency department visits. Know what your deductible is for you and for any others on your health plan. A little bit of planning goes a long way toward preventing insurance problems.

Let's review some of the basic information and terminology around insurance to help you understand better what that paperwork you receive in the mail means. This is also helpful in having a conversation with someone at either the billing department of your clinic or with your insurance carrier. It is not a bad idea to hold onto the "EOB" or Explanation of Benefits report that you receive in the mail or e-mail from your insurance company after a service, hospitalization or appointment. It can help you navigate and work through how charges were filed, what was covered and what your portion of the bill is. If you have any questions, this is especially helpful to reference when you are discussing your bill with the insurance provider or a local clinic or health system billing department.

Quick Reference of Frequently Used Insurance Terminology

Allowed Amount: The maximum amount a plan will pay for a covered health care service. May also be called "eligible expense," "payment allowance," or "negotiated rate." If your provider charges more than the plan's allowed amount, you may have to pay the difference.

Annual Deductible Combined: Usually in Health Savings Account (HSA) eligible plans, the total amount that family members on a plan must pay out-of-pocket for health care or prescription drugs before the health plan begins to pay.

Annual Limit: A cap on the benefits your insurance company will pay in a year while you're enrolled in a particular health insurance plan. These caps are sometimes placed on particular services such as prescriptions or hospitalizations. Annual limits may be placed on the dollar amount of covered services or on the number of visits that will be covered for a particular service. After an annual limit is reached, you must pay all associated health care costs for the rest of the year.

Appeal: A request for your health insurance company or the Health Insurance Marketplace to review a decision that denies a benefit or payment.

- If you don't agree with a decision made by the Marketplace, you may be able to file an appeal. Small businesses can also appeal Small Business Health Options Program (SHOP) decisions.
- If your health plan refuses to pay a claim or ends your coverage, you have the right to appeal the decision and have it reviewed by a third party.

Balance Billing: When a provider bills you for the difference between the provider's charge and the allowed amount. For example, if the provider's charge is $100 and the allowed amount is $70, the provider may bill you for the remaining $30. A preferred provider may not balance bill you for covered services.

Co-Insurance: The percentage of costs of a covered health care service you pay (20%, for example) after you've paid your deductible. Generally speaking, plans with lower monthly premiums have higher co-insurance, and plans with higher monthly premiums have lower co-insurance. In-network co-insurance usually costs you less than out-of-network co-insurance.

- Let's say your health insurance plan's allowed amount for an office visit is $100 and your coinsurance is 20%. If you've paid your deductible: You pay 20% of $100, or $20. The insurance company pays the rest.

  If you haven't met your deductible: You pay the full allowed amount, $100.

- Example of coinsurance with high medical costs

  Let's say the following amounts apply to your plan and you need a lot of treatment for a serious condition. Allowable costs are $12,000.

Deductible: $3,000. Coinsurance: 20%. Out-of-pocket maximum: $6,850. You'd pay all of the first $3,000 (your deductible). You'll pay 20% of the remaining $9,000, or $1,800 (your coinsurance). So, your total out-of-pocket costs would be $4,800 — your $3,000 deductible plus your $1,800 coinsurance. If your total out-of-pocket costs reach $6,850, you'd pay only that amount, including your deductible and coinsurance. The insurance company would pay for all covered services for the rest of your plans year.

Co-payment (copays): A fixed amount ($20, for example) you pay for a covered health care service after you've paid your deductible. Co-payments can vary for different services within the same plan, like drugs, lab tests, and visits to specialists. Generally, plans with lower monthly premiums have higher copayments. Plans with higher monthly premiums usually have lower co-payments. In-network co-payments usually are less than out-of-network co-payments.

- Let's say your health insurance plan's allowable cost for a doctor's office visit is $100. Your co-payment for a doctor visit is $20. If you've paid your **deductible:** You pay $20, usually at the time of the visit. If you haven't met your deductible: You pay $100, the full allowable amount for the visit.

Coordination of Benefits: A way to figure out who pays first when 2 or more health insurance plans are responsible for paying the same medical claim.

Deductible: The amount you pay for covered health care services before your insurance plan starts to pay. With a $2,000 deductible, for example, you pay the first $2,000 of covered services yourself. Generally, plans with lower monthly premiums have higher deductibles. Plans with higher monthly premiums usually have lower deductibles.

- After you pay your deductible, you usually pay only a co-payment or co-insurance for covered services. Your insurance company pays the rest. Many plans pay for certain services, like a checkup or disease management programs before you've met your deductible. Check your plan details. All Marketplace health plans pay the full cost of certain preventive benefits even before you meet your deductible.

- Some plans have separate deductibles for certain services, like prescription drugs.

- Family plans often have both an individual deductible, which applies to each person, and a family deductible, which applies to all family members.

Lifetime Limit: A cap on the total lifetime benefits you may get from your insurance company. An insurance company may impose a total lifetime dollar limit on benefits (like a $1 million lifetime cap) or limits on specific benefits (like a $200,000 lifetime cap on organ transplants or one gastric bypass per lifetime) or a combination of the two. After a lifetime limit is reached, the insurance plan will no longer pay for covered services.

Medically Necessary: Health care services or supplies needed to diagnose or treat an illness, injury, condition, disease or its symptoms and that meet accepted standards of medicine.

Network: The facilities, providers and suppliers your health insurer or plan has contracted with to provide health care services.

Network Plan: A health plan that contracts with doctors, hospitals, pharmacies, and other health care providers to provide members of the plan with services and supplies at a discounted price.

Out-of-Pocket Costs: Your expenses for medical care that aren't reimbursed by insurance. Out-of-pocket costs include deductibles, co-insurance, and co-payments for covered services plus all costs for services that aren't covered.

Out-of-Pocket Maximum/Limit: The most you have to pay for covered services in a plan year. After you spend this amount on deductibles, co-payments, and co-insurance for in-network care and services, your health plan pays 100% of the costs of covered benefits.

The out-of-pocket limit doesn't include:

- Your monthly premiums

- Anything you spend for services your plan doesn't cover.

- Out-of-network care and services.

- Costs above the allowed amount for a service that a provider may charge.

Other Useful Healthcare Related Terminology can be found in Appendix A.

TIPS:

-Familiarize yourself with what your insurance policy covers and what your payment will be: co-payment, co-insurance, allowed amount, deductible are good items to start with.

-Consider filing your EOB statement from your insurance company until all claims are paid.

(The above terminology is taken from https://www.healthcare.gov/glossary accessed April 18, 2023. Further terminology available online)

Chapter 14
Aging, End of Life Issues and Death

(AKA: Let's not talk about that….)

Aging

We live in a society that values youth and vitality. We spend absurd amounts of money chasing it: plastic surgery, Botox, personal trainers, supplements, and the list goes on. This is not a judgement on any of these, and I have personally participated in these pursuits as well. In the US we work intensely *(often leaving vacation time unused-768 million days of PTO in 2018!)*[1] when we're young and look to retire with the hope of spending our later lives doing all the things that we didn't get to do when we were younger.

The irony is when we get older and ready to enact all of those plans our health often interferes, and we find ourselves with an aging body, limitations, or serious health issues in ourselves and friends and family members. We relegate our older citizens to nursing homes, assisted living facilities and try not to think too much about how that will be us one day. I consider our views on aging one of the fatal flaws of our modern society.

In the past and in other cultures, we understood the value of the accumulated life experiences of those older than us. We're not talking about wisdom, as this is not really a function of aging and can be found in all ages, but experience. I have seen solutions proposed for a problem within a clinic only to have older providers in the group relate they had tried the same approach in the past and were able to relay the issues they encountered and why it didn't work. We were then able to contribute and come up with a new solution instead of recreating the same scenario and having to experience the same failures. The philosopher George Santayana said, *"Those who cannot remember the past are condemned to repeat it.*" We usually think of this in terms of the grand scale of global history, but I wonder how much of the mundane daily aspects of our lives reflect this, at home, at work, in relationships and in our daily decisions. Maybe we recreate the same issues when we discount the input of those who have *"been there, done that."* Not to say that a fresh perspective is not of value as we age it is easy to become more rigid in our beliefs and how we position ourselves. If something works, we can choose to decide this is the only way to do it. There is a value in the perspective of someone who is not entrenched in a particular method. The key is understanding the value of each side and drawing from each in a collaborative effort.

In relation to health, it is important that we shift our views on aging. It is an inevitable part of our journey. Resisting utilizes time and energy better spent on enjoying the present in any way we can. Resistance automatically says aging is not ok and to be dealt with like any other medical problem. ***It is not a medical***

problem. I have encountered many patients in their 80's and 90's living full, joyful lives, while other patients in their 30's are unhealthy and unhappy. Successful seniors can choose to live within each day and what it offers. This is not to discount attention to good nutrition, regular exercise, healthy relationships and stress management, as these all combine to support healthy aging; the healthier your body, the easier it can be to enjoy being older. If you can't walk because your knees hurt too badly or you are too short of breath related to lung disease, enjoying being older or life at any age is much more of a challenge.

The unfortunate reality is many of us don't pay attention when our bodies subtly, or not so subtly, tell us that something is off, and we wait until our bodies scream at us to change our lifestyle. It is hard to unwind at 70 all of the issues your body has been telling you for the past 30-plus years. The key is not just prioritizing healthy nutrition, exercise, stress management, but doing all of these things in order to support the optimal functioning of your body. The goal is health, not just looking younger, more sculpted, slimmer, and the list goes on. And consider being kinder to yourself: practice looking in the mirror and telling yourself how amazing you are and quit picking out every wrinkle and extra fold and defect. It does take practice. I know, as it is an ongoing struggle for me, but the results of your effort can directly impact your mental health. It can be liberating to let go of the way in which many of us have spent out lives, living out what others say we are expected to do, look like and act like. Be who you really are. Maybe we could take a note from earlier cultures who have embraced the value of the wise elders and crones, wrinkles and all.

End of life issues

Just like aging is inevitable, the failure of our bodies to support us is also inevitable. It may be the cancer that has spread despite treatment, the kidney failure where we don't tolerate dialysis anymore, or the dementia that tells us we're full as we slowly starve.

The question is not whether our bodies will fail, the question is how.

It is crucial that each of us considers this and has discussions with our families on what we want and don't want. Please don't assume that everyone knows. I have unfortunately too often witnessed arguments between family members who all thought they knew what a patient wanted, right up until something happened and they realized they didn't. What a terrible time for division among family. Sit down with who will participate in making those decisions for you if and when you cannot; your spouse, family member, close friend or someone you designate as medical power of attorney. There are several designations and the laws can vary from state to state on who has the power to make health care decisions for you if you cannot. You may want every possible thing done to prolong your life (Full Code), no intervention at all (DNR: do not resuscitate), only interventions to keep you comfortable (Comfort Care), and there are others. They each tell the medical system to behave in a certain way when your body fails. We will make sure that your wishes are upheld if you have completed this process. If your family member wants things you don't, we will respect your wishes if you have made them clear. It is imperative that you make sure that a copy is in your chart, that anyone involved has a copy and you have a copy. I have often thought this is such a huge event in our lives, and yet many of us devote little to no time to it. Of course, these recommendations hold true for everyone, despite their age. We don't know when we will need it and we have all heard the emotional stories of people dying unexpectedly or at a young age. It is fascinating that I have only had a handful of patients over the years come in for an appointment just to discuss these issues and clarify what each type of designation means. If we can make an appointment to discuss the best treatment for a sinus infection, surely this deserves the same level of attention, no matter what our age.

Transition between hospitalization and "Home"

An older family member of mine was a functioning independent individual until hospitalization for an acute medical issue. While the issue was addressed and controlled, the peripheral effects of being hospitalized and ill, even for a short time, were dramatic. This is unfortunately a common occurrence in patients who are older. They had loss of stable walking, confusion and difficulty with the activities of daily life (ADL's). They went to a rehabilitation hospital after discharge from the acute care hospital and got better, but not back to baseline. They wanted to go home from there, and most of us would want the same. Home is where you feel comfortable and is indeed where healing can more effectively take place. But. There's always that "but." If a patient is not ready to really go home and function well, home may not be the best option. My family member went home and did improve, but not at the pace that would have occurred with more consistent and intensive assistance, and the trajectory was not toward recovering previous levels of functioning. So, family members then had to begin the laborious process of getting them admitted into a rehabilitation facility. We then had to have further discussions on next steps including evaluating other placement options if being independent at home was no longer an option.

This transition between hospitalization and home is a significant challenge for both parents and families. There are several options to help with this transition. Home health can provide much needed care to support recovery at home after hospitalizations and allow patients to go home sooner. They can provide IV medications, physical therapy, medication review, home assistance needs and others. They can also be a way to treat a patient at home for a minor issue that otherwise would require hospitalization. However, there are limits to what type of services a patient qualifies for, and on the duration of service. These limits are not set by your provider and they have no control over their implementation.

Skilled nursing facilities (also known as SNF's) are a common transition between hospitalization and back to the patient's usual living situation, either home or a living facility. They provide 24 nursing services similar to being in a hospital, allowing a patient to recover from an illness, surgery, injury or worsened chronic illness. For example, if your elderly mother is hospitalized for pneumonia but has lost strength and mobility while there, she could be discharged to a skilled nursing facility to be monitored while receiving physical therapy, respiratory therapy to recover back to baseline breathing and strength. This is a type of rehabilitation and is doctor supervised, but the amount of services is usually one to two hours per day. Providers are available but are only generally required to see patients once every thirty days, relying on reports from the nursing staff. Patients may be confused because these facilities are often housed within a wing of a hospital or within a nursing home, but they are not the same as in-patient hospital care or a nursing home. There is a limit to the number of days that insurance will pay for a stay in a skilled nursing facility. Patients who do not improve within their allotted days require ongoing care may have to enter a nursing home for prolonged recovery needs.

In contrast, in-patient rehabilitation facilities or hospitals are more intensive, providing more hours of services per day and providers see patients several times a week. Stays are generally shorter than skilled nursing facilities, 16 days as opposed to 28 days.

There are other types of long-term care facilities such as long-term rehabilitation facilities, but these are usually more specialized for long term issues such as ventilator (breathing machine) patients.

Death

We surely do not like talking about this topic, but the one guarantee in life is that you will die. In our culture we typically avoid discussions on death, but in other cultures it is talked about more openly. Because there is so much fear around death, it carries a huge emotional charge for most of us. In western countries death frequently occurs in hospitals or other health-care settings, so the act of dying is frequently kept hidden from public view.[2] COVID however brought death front and center, and findings of a recent study showed that COVID-19 anxiety is positively related to fear of death, suggesting that individuals with higher COVID-19 anxiety were more likely to experience fear of death and vice versa.[3]

The uncertainty around death is just something we do not tolerate well, so we try to mold it into something more acceptable. How many times have you heard the comment at an open casket funeral that *"They look just like they're sleeping."* Consider why we try to make a deceased person look like they're really just resting in a casket. Again, not a condemnation or judgement but an observation, and everyone deals with death in the way that seems best to them. There are so many views on what happens after we die, and I have seen heated arguments on this very topic both in hospital rooms and at social dinners. It would seem logical that whether you believe in Heaven, reincarnation, or a change to just energy, this process should not induce fear, as it is a universal truth. However, we just don't like the unknown, and even belief in an afterlife doesn't negate the fear. One systematic analysis of multiple international studies showed only those that are "very religious" (religious behavior driven by "true belief") and atheists enjoy the least anxiety around dying.[4] It is interesting that we avoid even saying someone is dead. We use words like "transitioning", "passed", "passed on", "with God", "in a better place" etc. Again, we clearly don't like the unknown and death is the biggest unknown of all.

I bring this up to ask you to consider your thoughts and feelings on death. We go to classes to practice for childbirth, we have a rehearsal dinner to practice getting married, we take practice tests for important examinations, we practice our interview techniques before we interview for the job that we want. *Why don't we practice or plan for the one guarantee that affects us all?* Few of us have even thought about, much less planned how we want our family or friends to honor our death. Is it a celebration with music, dancing and recounting of stories? Is it somber? Do you want a casket and embalming, or cremation? Did you want something different: buried in a mushroom coffin, buried with a tree planted over you, cremation in water (aquamation), sky burials where vultures eat your body, donation to a body farm for research, donation to science for research, sea burial, human composting? You can even turn your loved one's ashes into diamonds of all things. Keeping the idea of death locked up and taboo only serves to enhance the fear we have around it. Psychologists and therapists use "exposure therapy" as one way to address fear, where they create a safe environment in which to "expose" individuals to the things they fear and avoid. Maybe we should talk more freely about death to lessen the fear, starting with the people closest to us. If you are looking for community support, there are even "Death Cafes" where groups gather in person and online to "eat cake, drink tea and discuss death" (https://deathcafe.com)[5]. Life is full of initiations: birth, first kiss, marriage, first job, and yes, death. We should bring death out of the closet and normalize our final initiation in this lifetime, whatever that may be.

Keep in mind that you are not on your own as you navigate this. A lawyer can help you understand your rights, and many local agencies on aging and health systems have resources to assist you with documenting your preferences on illness, death and dying. Talk to your primary provider about your preferences and ask for resources.

Consider that The Dalai Lama, when asked what surprised him most about humanity, he said:

"Man.
Because he sacrifices his health in order to make money.
Then he sacrifices money to recuperate his health.
And then he is so anxious about the future that he does not enjoy the present;
the result being that he does not live in the present or the future;
he lives as if he is never going to die, and then dies having never really lived."

TIPS

-Have an open discussion with your family or caretakers on your personal wishes of how you wish any serious life-threatening illness and your death and dying managed.

-Document your preferences and provide caretakers and family members with a copy.

-Make sure that you, your family or caregivers, and EHR if applicable, has a copy of your preferences.

References

1.https://www.ustravel.org/sites/default/files/media_root/document/Paid%20Time%20Off%20Trends%20Fact%20Sheet.pdf?utm_source=MagnetMail&utm_medium=email&utm_content=8%2E15%2E19%2DPress%2DVacation%20Days%20Release&utm_campaign=pr)

2. Muramatsu, N., Hoyem, R. L., Yin, H., & Campbell, R. T. (2008). Place of death among older Americans: Does state spending on home- and community-based services promote home death? *Medical Care, 46*(8), 829–838. https://doi.org/10.1097/MLR.0b013e3181791a79

3. Bulut, M.B. Relationship between COVID-19 anxiety and fear of death: the mediating role of intolerance of

uncertainty among a Turkish sample. *Curr Psychol* (2022). https://doi.org/10.1007/s12144-022-03281-x

4. Jonathan Jong, Robert Ross, Tristan Philip, Si-Hua Chang, Naomi Simons & Jamin Halberstadt (2018) The religious correlates of death anxiety: a systematic review and meta-analysis, Religion, Brain & Behavior, 8:1, 4-20, DOI: 10.1080/2153599X.2016.1238844

5. https://deathcafe.com/

Chapter 15
The Personal Accountability Factor

(AKA: At least half of this is on you!)

We've discussed multiple issues behind the scenes that can impact the quality of your healthcare. Many of these can significantly have a negative or positive impact on your overall health when you encounter them in the course of your care. **Going to see your provider does not equal health!** Your provider can be a resource of information and recommendations but cannot exercise for you or take your medications for you. We haven't talked about the impact of your choices on your health. We all have the right to choose how we wish to live our lives, and to determine how we wish to manage our healthcare. We also have the right to experience the consequences of those choices. I have been yelled at several times by frightened patients or family members who blamed me for a condition that had progressed by the time it was diagnosed. The tests to evaluate for it were ordered months before when the patient first came in, but life got in the way and they didn't prioritize it. It is difficult to accept when we are at fault, especially when our choices impact us directly. The *"shoulda, woulda, coulda"* scenario is unfortunately one that we have all encountered in our lives in some way. It is especially painful when it occurs with our health.

Stand up for your health and care for your body. We often get overwhelmed thinking that to have an impact we must meet the guidelines for how much exercise, how much sugar and fat to limit, how much of this and how much of that. The truth is that small changes can translate into significant impacts on our health. For example, a recent meta-analysis showed that standing intermittently can impact glucose levels, and light walking (2-5 minutes) after eating can reduce both glucose and insulin levels.[1] Both are a big win for your health. If you are older and have prediabetes, going for a

15-minute walk (not a jog or power walking) after eating meals is as good as a single 45-minute walk.[2] Don't get caught up in which is the "right" diet as <u>ANY</u> efforts at reducing processed foods, adding fruits, vegetables and fiber can impact your health without requiring you to rethink your entire diet. Consider a basic change such as stopping or reducing sugary beverages, as intake of added sugars in drinks promotes weight gain and is linked to Type 2 diabetes, cardiovascular disease, and gout. Put more colorful fruits and vegetables on your plate while cutting back on white bread and refined starch sides; choose whole grains and whole-grain foods over refined; snack on nuts or fruit instead of pretzels or potato chips if hunger strikes between meals; and add beans and lentils to soups, salads, and side dishes. Consider that the intention behind what you do might be as important as the action itself. Find interventions that make you feel empowered and not deprived.

Changing behavior is hard, and small steps are more likely to lead to sustainable and manageable change.[3] When there are so many different diets, exercise plans, and suggestions on how to lose weight and be "healthy" you can be sure that no one has the "one real" answer. Some methods work for one person and a completely different method works for others. You can even find "intuitive eating coaches" to help you understand what might resonate best with you. Explore what works for you and what you can stick with. There is no one right way, and being consistent with your efforts may be more important than the type of intervention. The best dietary or exercise practice in the world doesn't matter if you cannot maintain it. Science is at the cusp of the ability to guide us individually on what might be our most effective dietary and exercise efforts. Until these are easily accessible, any efforts toward a healthier lifestyle count. Please don't get caught up in the idea that it's too late. It is never too late to intervene. Start now to take care of your body and improve your health!

Also, let's not ignore the proverbial elephant in the room: **stress**. Our bodies are designed to manage intermittent stress quite effectively; whether a real tiger or the metaphorical one at work or home. The problem is that we are NOT designed to remain in a constant state of stress – the tiger eats us or we get away: either way the stress ends. The constant stress state that most of us live in here in the United States creates havoc with our health. A survey released by the American Psychological Association in 2022 found that an alarming proportion of adults reported that stress has an impact on their day-to-day functioning, with more than a quarter (27%) saying that most days they are so stressed they can't function.[4]

What an alarming statistic! Remember, you don't have to quit your job or leave your family or otherwise turn your life upside down to effect change. Just like with diet and exercise, small interventions can have a measurable impact. Consider integrating a breathing exercise into your day. An example is the 4-7-8 technique that Dr. Andrew Weil at the University of Arizona Center for Integrative Medicine recommends and is an easy way to help reduce the stress response. Breathe in through your nose for a 4 count, hold for a 7 count and breathe out through your mouth for an 8 count. This is just one example and if this one doesn't work for you, there are numerous other breathing exercises you can explore. Meditation *(don't wince or roll your eyes as my family does!)* is effective and does not have to be sitting on a cushion creating more stress from trying to quiet your mind. You can do walking meditation, chant, dance to music, or whatever makes you feel more connected, relaxed and grounded. Consider mindfulness, a type of meditation in which you focus on being intensely aware of what you're sensing and feeling in the moment, without interpretation or judgment. Mindfulness practices can be as simple as intermittently closing your eyes and focusing on your breath as it travels in and out of your body; stopping an activity and noticing what is around you and how your body feels; looking at the horizon for a few minutes. Look up mindfulness and you might be surprised at the robust research data supporting its impact.

Consider what <u>you could do that resonates with you</u> to support your health. Your provider is a resource but cannot function as your health coach – we would love to but reality is there is not time to do this for you. What occurs in an 15 to 20 minute appointment with your provider does not compare to the impact that the choices you make during the rest of your life will. The take-home is all of us can find a way to integrate small changes into our busy lives to improve our health, and it's never too late to make that change. We just have to care about and prioritize caring for ourselves as much as we do about others, our jobs and all the other things in our lives that demand our attention.

TIPS

-Consider one small dietary change, and after you have incorporated it into your routine, add another.

-Consider standing frequently for a few minutes if you have a sedentary job and going for a light walk after meals

-Consider implementing a type of breathing or mindfulness practice into your day – whatever works for you.

References

1. Buffey, A.J., Herring, M.P., Langley, C.K. *et al.* The Acute Effects of Interrupting Prolonged Sitting Time in Adults with Standing and Light-Intensity Walking on Biomarkers of Cardiometabolic Health in Adults: A Systematic Review and Meta-analysis. *Sports Med* **52**,

1765–1787 (2022). https://doi.org/10.1007/s40279-022-01649-4

2. Loretta DiPietro, Andrei Gribok, Michelle S. Stevens, Larry F. Hamm, William Rumpler; Three 15-min Bouts of Moderate Postmeal Walking Significantly Improves 24-h Glycemic Control in Older People at Risk for Impaired Glucose Tolerance. *Diabetes Care* 1 October 2013; 36 (10): 3262–3268.

3. https://nutrition.tufts.edu/news/small-changes-can-have-big-impact-health. Accessed April 18, 2023.

4. *https://www.apa.org/news/press/releases/stress/2022/concerned-future-inflation accessed 5/10/23.*

Chapter 16
The Disconnect

(aka "This isn't freaking working!")

I used to say and think that the United States has the best medical care in the world. We do have amazing technology and treatments that continue to astound me. But as with any system, the value of something is measured by its large-scale overall outcomes, and compared to our peer countries we are not effectively utilizing our resources in healthcare. According to the Commonwealth Fund publication *U.S. Health Care from a Global Perspective*[1] we find the following information:

-Health care spending, both per person and as a share of GDP, continues to be far higher in the United States than in other high-income countries. Yet the U.S. is the only country that doesn't have universal health coverage.

-The U.S. has the lowest life expectancy at birth, the highest death rates for avoidable or treatable conditions, the highest maternal and infant mortality, and among the highest suicide rates.

-The U.S. has the highest rate of people with multiple chronic conditions and an obesity rate nearly twice the OECD average. (The Organization for Economic Co-operation and Development (OECD) is a unique forum where the governments of 37 democracies with market-based economies collaborate to develop policy standards to promote sustainable economic growth)

-Americans see physicians less often than people in most other countries and have among the lowest rate of practicing physicians and hospital beds per 1,000 population.

One could study the "whys" behind these statistics for years and not find one single answer, as the causes are many. Some of this is due to system issues, some due to collective societal issues and some due to personal accountability issues, both on the side of patients and providers. One of the current concerns I have perceived relates to trying to reduce health into data points and running it strictly as a business. It sounds great on paper: if the data says this, we go down this algorithm. If it says something different, we use another algorithm. We have moved the decision point so far up the administrative chain that the data is all there is, and much of the humanity needed has been lost.

Data is important and helps as a guide but the complexities of health cannot be truly weighed and measured with simple spreadsheets.

When your front-line workers are asked to operate from a position of compassion and care that the system wants, but yet every decision at an administrative level is made without prioritizing those variables, how can a system not fail? It results in our current mentality of burnout for front line workers and frustration and distrust from patients. The situations created encourage everyone to default back to *"I have to do what I have to do to take care of me and mine."* Now we have been effectively isolated into individuals fighting with each other for scraps under the table while the elite few determine from on high which scraps they are willing to throw. It is the age-old tactic of keeping everyone divided and fighting because if they join into a collective they are a threat to the ones in control.

This sounds rather medieval and surely cannot occur in a modern society you say. Consider the example of the inability of many "well meaning" people who are in positions of power within the healthcare system to see their place in this problem. For example (and there are many), a CEO of a health care system in April 2020 (we all remember this frightening time) announced a hiring freeze and asked employees to voluntarily take leave without pay, use personal time off or reduce their normal work week; saying the hospital was also considering mandating workers to use their paid time off, mandatory leave without pay and other steps. One week later the management had their 2019 incentive bonuses deposited into their account and had been notified of this in late March. The CEO apologized for the "timing" of the bonuses but defended them as keeping the executives at the midpoint of compensation range compared to their counterparts across the country.[2]

I am sure that the front-line workers at that hospital didn't see it the same way. How egregious that this is seems obvious looking in from the outside, but humans are interesting creatures in our ability to perceive events to fit our narratives. And situations like these are ongoing and heard in informal conversations at gatherings of providers and health care workers across the country. It's a great example of the disconnect that has occurred as healthcare became an "industry", and I perceive that many of our current issues began when we transitioned to health as a business commodity.

I clearly remember attending Grand Rounds when I was an Internal Medicine resident many years ago. Grand Rounds is a lecture series for providers covering new topics, updates etc. and a foundational educational experience at most academic institutions, and some non-academic hospitals as well. The Chair of Medicine, a brilliant physician and patient advocate, gave a talk on HMO's (Health Maintenance Organizations), which was a new entity at the time. He was upset at what he called the demise of healthcare, and I clearly remember thinking how dramatic he was being. Little did I know I would vividly recall his lecture years later and reflect on what a prophet he was. He showed a slide from one HMO that referenced patients as customers and commented on what a profound change this was – shifting the entire dynamic from the complexity of the patient and provider relationship to a simple exchange of money for a service. No different that dropping your car off at a mechanic. He also was deeply concerned about providers being placed as "gatekeepers", meaning a patient had to have a provider refer them to access any specialist. Prior to this, patients could often ask for appointments with specialists directly, or be referred, but did not require the primary care provider to approve it. This set up the patient provider relationship as adversarial instead of being a team. If you disagreed with your provider about seeing a specialist as a patient you were upset, and sometimes rightly so. In this scenario, as a provider you had to justify to the system "why" you were referring a patient and at the same time assume responsibility for the adverse outcomes if you didn't. A nightmare for both patients and providers, and the beginning of the slow dissolution of the relationship. In retrospect, as with many issues in our society today, was the attack on this relationship intentional? A patient/provider team on the same page is powerful and a force to be dealt with. But if you can place them on opposite sides, you can play to the fears of each and further divide, allowing the power focus to remain higher up. *Does this sound familiar: politics, religious issues, etc.?*

As we try to shift the paradigm in healthcare maybe what we call each other should also be questioned. While the words consumer or customer supports the idea of the relationship as just a business transaction, our current terminology of "patient" could be improved. The term "provider" implies that we are providing you with health. We can provide you with the tools but we cannot provide the "health." And one definition of the word "patient" according to Merriam-Webster means *bearing pains or trials calmly or without complaining, manifesting forbearance under provocation or strain.* This sounds a lot like the actual experience of what many patients endure today. Maybe a better word would be "client", and there are many others to consider. Perhaps we could employ words that denote a more team centric approach to healthcare, with all parties clearly understanding their individual responsibilities to reach a common goal. The bottom line is we hope you understand from our perspective as your health care provider/manager/partner, our relationship is more than a simple exchange of money for services. We are privy to your successes, your failures, your family dramas, your heartbreaks, your pain and your joy. We celebrate and grieve with you. We are invested in your health and your life. The diminishment and in many cases loss of this personal relationship underlies much of provider frustration in our current system in primary care.

This frustration is also compounded by this shift to more of a business model on all levels, not just the provider/patient relationship. We as providers are expected to embody the values of caring, compassion and diligence but aren't rewarded when we do *(ie: our monthly performance report says we're just not meeting our percentile goal for seeing enough patients)*. We are encouraged to diligently complete all of our tasks behind the scenes with careful attention, and systems rely heavily on these qualities of diligence, caring and compassion to ensure that we do. They know that most of us feel deeply responsible for our patients' health. But again, there is little to no compensation for these qualities that the systems rely on. What you may not realize is being considered a customer or "covered life" reduces you again to a simple datapoint on a spreadsheet to systems who are trying to allocate resources. We receive our review of our "performance" of how we are doing within our systems on a regular basis and asked to switch gears from the compassionate provider to business minded professionals as we evaluate our personal data. What a disconnect: primary care providers are by nature mainly focused on our patients and optimizing their care but are then asked to turn that off and evaluate our performance as a business. This was an appropriate ask when physicians owned and ran their practices as a business, as they had control over and could directly allocate resources based on where they were needed at the time to optimize care among their patient population. They could look at a granular level where resources were spent and whether that spend was having the desired effect at a clinic level, and they were nimble enough to pivot as needed. Large systems do the same but the agility is lost and the amount of data too cumbersome and impersonal to be effective at an individual patient level.

To summarize, the paradox for providers currently is we are asked to effectively think of our clinic as a business and be responsible for outcomes, but we have little to no control over the variables that impact the outcomes.

In essence, compassion, personal attention and emotional support are things that are difficult to measure, so are for the most part downplayed or ignored completely as a measure of success by a business entity.

But these qualities are the bedrock foundation of caring for patients.

References

1.https://www.commonwealthfund.org/publications/issue-briefs/2023/jan/us-health-care-global-perspective-2022. Accessed April 18, 2023.

2.https://www.cbsnews.com/colorado/news/coronavirus-denver-health-bonus-ceo-pay-cuts/. Accessed April 18, 2023.

Chapter 17
Reflections on Health

(AKA: Outside the box is not always a bad place to be!)

Ok, we reviewed the logistics and issues around our current healthcare system: the problems, work arounds, etc. All of this to support your goals of optimizing your health. But what is health? Oxford Languages says it is a noun with the following meanings: *the state of being free from illness or injury; a person's mental or physical condition.* I much prefer the World Health Organizations definition: *Health is a state of complete physical, mental and social well-being and not merely the absence of disease or infirmity.* This definition honors the idea that what one individual considers health may vary drastically from another individual. Neither are right or wrong.

As the definition of health is not a rigid construct, the optimal management of an individual patient is also not rigid and set in stone. The old paternalistic approach of telling a patient what to do has been replaced with discussions with patients on how best to manage their medical issue. Therapies such as acupuncture that were once regarded as unproven and "fringe" by medical academia are now a part of routine recommendations for patients. We now have studies showing the effectiveness of this intervention. Supplements and botanicals that were considered to be the purview of the uninformed now have data and are commonly recommended by mainstream providers (my family member just told me that her orthopedic physician told her of the benefits of turmeric). It is gratifying to see that we as a medical community are opening up more and more to what is considered non-traditional approaches. Patients now have more options and more providers willing to consider alternative interventions. But it is important to recognize the appropriate time and place for traditional and alternative therapies. There are those, both patients and providers, who refuse to consider alternative therapies. There are others who refuse to utilize traditional therapies. There is a place for each, and choosing to completely avoid one or the other can limit your options and outcomes.

STAY OPEN.

The scientific method says that we must come up with an idea then prove it with testing. This means that we verify in the research lab that something is credible or "real" before we accept it. This approach has resulted in huge advancements in medicine and improving patient lives and is the backbone of science. Traditionally, any treatment or intervention that was outside the scientific method was not considered valid, but we are slowly starting to recognize that not everything fits into this rigid model. There are interventions that have been used for thousands of years in some cultures that we are just now beginning to apply the scientific method to with positive results, with subsequent integration into more mainstream practice. Practitioners who have been utilizing these ancient therapies often roll their eyes and say, *"Well of course they work – I've used them successfully for years."* So yes, the scientific method is important but it is not the only model that we can choose to use. Sometimes the intervention, process or finding precedes our ability to measure and quantify it. For example: in the book *Stealing Fire* by Steven Kotler and Jamie Wheal, the authors discuss how Google and the Navy Seals looked for specific qualities in who they selected that had nothing to do with traditional accepted measures of what an ideal candidate was at that time. They just knew it was an intangible "something" that resulted in a desired outcome in their final selections. Years have gone by and now we have developed the ability to actually measure and train for some of these qualities. So, what seemed like so much craziness then is now considered more "real" and acceptable.

All of this seems reminiscent of how more primitive cultures viewed technology when first introduced to it: it must be magic! There just wasn't a knowledge or experience foundation for these cultures to view it otherwise. I question whether we are similar to these primitive cultures in how we perceive some of the more fantastical findings that seem to be cropping up everywhere. Much is likely so much smoke and mirrors, but rather than completely rejecting all of it, it would seem more prudent to evaluate each with an open mind and see what unfolds. As an example, in the early 1990's the idea of carrying around a device roughly the size of your hand that could function as a phone, computer, camera, etc. was unheard of. Until it wasn't. A more "out there" example: water. Water is water, right? You can drink it, bathe in it, ski on a snowy slope of it, swim in it, put frozen cubes in your drinks to chill them, bask in a hot tub of water, etc. This pervasive common element has been with and around us since the beginning of time. Many don't know, however, that the French scientist Jacques Benveniste in 1988 published that water has a "memory", with his results confirmed by other independent labs in Italy, Canada and Israel at the time. The editor and chief of the scientific journal Nature, after initially publishing the results, refused to believe these astonishing findings and subsequently discredited the scientists involved. Michel Schiff later published a detailed description of the persecution of this scientist in his book, *The Memory of Water*. In it he denounces the dangers of censorship, stating *"the long history of scientific dogmatism shows that today's heresy could well become tomorrow's scientific truth."* The French virologist Luc Montagnier, who received in 1988 the Nobel Prize for his contribution to the discovery of the HIV virus, was also violently attacked when he resumed this experimental study of water memory.[1]

Hmmmm – this example is harder than the cell phone. Did you feel yourself reacting one way or the other? Can you lay aside any preconceived ideas and stay open to the possibility? Is it true or not? While intriguing, I cannot personally answer that and whether it is true is secondary. The goal is to not dismiss something just because it doesn't fit into what you thought was real, but to remain curious and explore for yourself whether it is credible. Remember that what we consider miracles may just be science that we can't understand yet.

In truth, anything that doesn't fit within our current agreed upon acceptance of what science is often is met with resistance, when it should be met with curiosity. Please understand that I am not suggesting that we abandon science and the scientific method. It is the anchor of our current medical system and has served us well. I only propose that it is not so easy to apply it to each and every treatment for an individual patient. We as providers, should always abide by that portion of the Hippocratic oath that all physicians swear to of "Primum Non Nocere (First Do No Harm)." This includes both not doing a harmful treatment AND not standing in the way of one that may work. In line with this tenet for example: If we think that the supplement that a patient is taking doesn't work and the benefit that the patient experiences is likely a "placebo" effect, but does no harm – does it matter if there is no formal scientific proof behind it? If you as the patient find relief with no harm, then it is of benefit. It <u>IS</u> our responsibility to help inform you as a patient of anything that could have negative consequences for your health, either by taking something unproven with known risks or refusing treatment. If you have appendicitis, we will recommend and believe that you should have urgent surgery, not take a botanical for it or do breathing exercises. However, you can refuse to have your appendix removed – it is your right. At the end of the day, patients have the right to weigh the pros and cons of any approach and make their own decisions. And as providers we have the right to refuse to facilitate treatments or interventions if we believe it is not in your best interest. We don't have to agree with every decision or intervention. And just as you can elect to seek out another provider if values don't align, we may also elect to ask you to see another provider for the same reasons. But unless your decisions harm others, we can and should support you in your journey of what you perceive as health.

I leave you with one final thought to consider on this: don't mix up the diagnosis and or name of your condition and the symptoms of the condition with what actually causes the condition. It's a dangerous circular logic that is easy to fall into. To paraphrase a quote from a lecture by Dr. Gabor Mate, author of several books on trauma: *"I have ADHD because I have impulse control, am distractible and tune out; and I have impulse control, am distractible and tune out because I have ADHD."* We have to get out our shovel and dig into what may underlie the problem. Maybe it is genetic, but maybe the main contributor to the condition is a lifestyle issue that is within our control to change. In fact, a study by researchers at Stanford School of Medicine recruited a set of patients who were tested for a gene that confers better exercise capacity and for a gene that can contribute to obesity. Baseline studies were obtained of each participant's exercise capacity and amount of the hormone related to eating that they produce after a meal. The participants were told the "results" of their tests but these "results" were randomly generated as positive or negative for each person. They were not necessarily the actual correct result for each. Then each participant underwent the same tests for exercise capacity and hormone production after a meal. What they found was astounding: some patients who actually had the gene for better exercise capacity but were told they didn't have the gene performed worse on the follow-up exercise testing. Some of those who actually DID have the gene for obesity associated with producing a lower amount of the hormone, but were told they didn't, produced higher levels on retesting.[2]) So genetics only provide a possibility for our health outcomes. Our perception of our risk and how we live our lives provides the actual healthy outcome. Our bodies communicate with us all the time, but we have to learn to listen. While your provider can assist you with this, much of the work falls to us as individuals to explore all our life experiences that may underlie our current symptoms.

References

1. Meessen, A. (2018) Water Memory Due to Chains of Nano-Pearls. *Journal of Modern Physics*, **9**, 2657-2724

2. Turnwald, B.P., Goyer, J.P., Boles, D.Z. *et al.* Learning one's genetic risk changes physiology independent of actual genetic risk. *Nat Hum Behav* **3**, 48–56 (2019). https://doi.org/10.1038/s41562-018-0483-4

CHAPTER 18
FOOD FOR THOUGHT

(AKA: IS THE GLASS HALF FULL OR HALF EMPTY?)

I hope that within these pages you have discovered what out-patient medicine looks like from the other side of the front desk and examination table. I hope you have opened a space for the struggle that your primary care provider (and all the clinical staff) go through daily in an attempt to care for you. Remember that you have the power to choose whether you react with anger (maybe justified or not) to a challenging situation that may occur or respond with more kindness and compassion in your interactions. The latter approach is much more work, but in the end benefits everyone involved, especially you. I have observed this ability to choose impact much more than just how you respond to having the appointment that you showed up for rescheduled when you arrive.

I have long been intrigued by this concept of choice. Throughout my career I have encountered patients who relay the problems they have, or have had, with their health and other life stressors and I internally recoil during their telling, thinking how can they endure such terrible things? As I prepare to extend a word of sympathy and compassion, I am shocked to observe them then shrug their shoulders and move on to telling me about other things in their lives. The terrible events are just a side dish in their life, not the main course. I used to think they were just not dealing with their issues, but as I followed them over time that just wasn't so. They were able to enjoy their lives and not let the "bad" overshadow the "good". I always then think to myself what is different about them that they can embrace the "good" and move the "bad" to a side to be dealt with but not focused on? That they manage to make the "problem" something that the management of is just worked into the fabric of their daily life. In contrast I have patients who encounter what from the outside looking in is a minor health issue or life stressor and their lives turn upside down and their entire focus becomes this issue or condition. This problem becomes the main course in their lives that everything revolves around. The quintessential glass half empty vs half full scenario. In my informal observations I haven't observed that education level, how dire the condition or event, family support or any consistent factor to predict or explain the response. Past trauma and mental health conditions certainly impacted responses but was not consistently present. Supportive factors in their lives seemed to help but didn't explain the difference in my many years of practice. In fact, I have seen patients who I would have squarely predicted to respond one way and yet they responded the opposite. Is it just how they perceive the issue, or choose to perceive the issue? When I ask the patients, who seem to be able to move on and thrive despite the issues, how they do it, one of the comments that I have heard often is something along the lines of *"Well I just choose to be happy and focus on the good things in my life"* (a paraphrased quote from one patient with cancer, the death of a child and other family members and financial crisis all in the same year). This seems so simplistic as to not be real, and almost a slap in the face to my patients who are struggling. But I have observed it over and over. It never fails to stop me in my tracks and make me rethink my response when I encounter a challenge in my life. Do the stories and projections about what occurs in our lives have such a great influence on how these things impact us? Maybe the way we choose to perceive it actually helps to craft the issue itself, as there is no doubt that stress worsens almost all medical conditions. Consider trauma, a huge issue in mental health, and something that most of us have encountered in our lives in some way, me included. Consider that residual trauma of any type is actually what happened INSIDE you as a result of what happened TO you, not the event itself. We can react to this definition with indignation as trauma immediately brings up images of terrible things happening to people and something that will always persist. But what if we choose to perceive this explanation of trauma another way: let's consider for a moment actually how encouraging this definition is. While we wouldn't have chosen the trauma and can't undo the event itself, if trauma is how we internalized and integrated the event, we can undo much of that with therapy and other techniques. We can choose to access therapies such as psychedelics that are available to help us "rewire" our brains to integrate our past wounding in a different way and reject the conditioning that these are only used by "drug abusers". We can choose to see our anxiety or depression symptoms as our body communicating with us, and not something external to us that is attacking our system. We can choose to reject processed foods and eat those that support our microbiome (the bacteria that live in our gut) so it can help optimize our mood *(yes, the brain and the gut talk – a lot).*

We can choose to practice mindfulness or meditate. We can choose to do yoga, tai chi, breathing exercises or any other practice that helps calm our nervous systems. We are not the victims that our culture often tells us we are. We can choose to remember we are amazing creatures capable of so much but have been indoctrinated from a young age to focus on our limitations and be the victims of a past depression or a future anxiety.

I ask you to reexamine the "why" behind your thoughts and actions. Are they based on YOUR beliefs and views, or that of your parents, society, educational systems, social media, a friend or some other entity that told you how to think? I encourage you to explore what options resonate with you when you consider healing and optimizing what you consider health. But remember that discernment is a critical tool in this journey, and one that we don't spend enough time utilizing. There is always someone caught up in chasing money and profit by preying on people who are desperately seeking answers or struggling. Just because you read it does not make it true. Just because it was posted on social media does not make it a fact. The truth is becoming harder and harder to sort out from the misinformation that is everywhere.

Being "open" to new ideas does not mean accepting every extreme therapy or idea you find. It does not mean discarding ideas just because they are traditional or mainstream, nor accepting them for the same reason. Do your research and be mindful of your resources for information. And it's okay to be wrong and to change your mind if you find new information. Choose to be open to new ideas but retain your right to question everything. While in matters of health, your health care provider is a resource, but they are an imperfect one, and your thoughts, your actions and your intention are the key to your well-being. Remember that health is an active process, not a passive one: no one can "give" **you** health, least of all a health care provider struggling themself.

Finally, don't let the "powers that be" convince you that you are separate from anyone, whether that someone is the clinic scheduler, your provider, the person with different political views, different religion or skin color. We all look the same underneath, we are all walking the same earth, and we are all struggling with something (no matter how it looks on the outside). We are all worthy of compassion and kindness (offering it to yourself MOST of all).

In parting, I share with you the thoughts of the Zen Buddhist monk Thich Nhat Hanh: *"People usually consider walking on water or in thin air a miracle. But I think the real miracle is not to walk either on water or in thin air, but to walk on earth. Every day we are engaged in a miracle which we don't even recognize: a blue sky, white clouds, green leaves, the black, curious eyes of a child – our own two eyes. All is a miracle."* [1.]

It took me far too many years to realize the simple unacknowledged miracle that I and my patients represent. An awake and aware patient and provider team is capable of much magic, and I know this from personal experience. I have cried with my patients and celebrated with them. The countless encounters, even the hard ones, I have had with my patients over many years opens my heart even as I write this. Being a part of your lives has been one of the great joys in my life, and I hope I helped all of you in some way. My greatest wish is that all of you choose to be the miracle that you are, starting today. I offer this book as a tool to help empower you within our current system until we can reimagine and reform healthcare. Until we can become partners in true healing and not just purveyors and consumers of goods from a broken system.

References

1. The Miracle of Mindfulness: An Introduction to the Practice of Meditation

Appendix A:

Other Useful Healthcare Related Terminology:

Accountable Care Organization: A group of health care providers who give coordinated care. Chronic disease management with the goal of improving the quality of patient care. Payment is tied to achieving health care quality metrics and outcomes.

Benefits: The health care items or services covered under a health insurance plan. Covered benefits and excluded services are defined in the health insurance plan's coverage documents. In Medicaid or CHIP, covered benefits and excluded services are defined in state program rules.

Cafeteria Plan: A cafeteria plan is a separate written plan maintained by an employer for employees that meets the specific requirements and regulations of Section 125 of the Internal Revenue Code. It provides participants with an opportunity to receive certain benefits on a pretax basis. Participants in a cafeteria plan must be permitted to choose from at least one taxable benefit (such as cash) and one qualified benefit.

Care Coordination: The organization of your treatment across several health care providers. Medical homes and

Accountable Care Organizations are two common ways to coordinate care.

Catastrophic Care Plan: Health plans that meet all of the requirements applicable to other Qualified Health Plans (QHPs) but don't cover any benefits other than 3 primary care visits per year before the plan's deductible is met. The premium amount you pay each month for health care is generally lower than for other QHPs, but the out-of-pocket costs for deductibles, co-payments, and co-insurance are generally higher. To qualify for a Catastrophic plan, you must be under 30 years old OR qualify for a "hardship" or "affordability" exemption if you're over 30.

Claim: A request for payment that you or your health care provider submits to your health insurer when you get items or services you think are covered.

COBRA: A federal law that may allow you to temporarily keep health coverage after your employment ends, you lose coverage as a dependent of the covered employee, or another qualifying event. If you elect COBRA (Consolidated Omnibus Budget Reconciliation Act) coverage, you pay 100% of the premiums, including the share the employer used to pay, plus a small administrative fee.

Cost sharing: The share of costs covered by your insurance that you pay out of your own pocket. This term generally includes deductibles, co-insurance, and co-payments, or similar charges, but it doesn't include premiums, balance billing amounts for non-network providers, or the cost of non-covered services. Cost sharing in Medicaid and CHIP also includes premiums.

Dependent: A child or other individual for whom a parent, relative, or other person may claim a personal exemption tax deduction. Under the Affordable Care Act, individuals may be able to claim a premium tax credit to help cover the cost of coverage for themselves and their dependents.

Donut Hole (Medicare Prescription Drug): Most plans with Medicare prescription drug coverage (Part D) have a coverage gap (called a "donut hole"). This means that after you and your drug plan have spent a certain amount of money for covered drugs, you have to pay all costs out-of-pocket for your prescriptions up to a yearly limit. Once you have spent up to the yearly limit, your coverage gap ends and your drug plan helps pay for covered drugs again.

Durable Medical Equipment (DME): Equipment and supplies ordered by a health care provider for everyday or extended use. Coverage for DME may include oxygen equipment, wheelchairs, crutches or blood testing strips for diabetics.

Emergency Medical Condition: An illness, injury, symptom or condition so serious that a reasonable person would seek care right away to avoid severe harm.

Emergency Services: Evaluation of an emergency medical condition and treatment to keep the condition from getting worse.

Employer Shared Responsibility Payment (ESRP): The Affordable Care Act requires certain employers with at least 50 full-time employees (or equivalents) to offer health insurance coverage to its full-time employees (and their dependents) that meets certain minimum standards set by the Affordable Care Act or to make a tax payment called the ESRP.

Exchange: Another term for the Health Insurance Marketplace˚, a service available in every state that helps individuals, families, and small businesses shop for and enroll in affordable medical insurance. The Marketplace is accessible through websites, call centers, and in-person assistance. When you fill out a Marketplace application, you'll find out if you qualify to save money when you enroll in a medical insurance plan. You'll also find out if you qualify for Medicaid and the Children's Health Insurance Program (CHIP). Whether you qualify for these programs depends on your expected income, household members, and other information.

Excluded Services: Health care services that your health insurance or plan doesn't pay for or cover.

Exemption: If you're 30 and older and want Catastrophic coverage, you must qualify for a "hardship" or "affordability" exemption. For plan years 2018 and earlier, other kinds of exemptions were granted based on certain hardships and life events, health coverage or financial status, membership in some groups, and other circumstances to avoid paying a fee that's no longer required.

External Review: A review of a plan's decision to deny coverage for or payment of a service by an independent third-party not related to the plan. If the plan denies an appeal, an external review can be requested. In urgent situations, an external review may be requested even if the internal appeals process isn't yet completed. External review is available when the plan denies treatment based on medical necessity, appropriateness, health care setting, level of care, or effectiveness of a covered benefit, when the plan determines that the care is experimental and/or investigational, or for rescissions of coverage. An external review either upholds the plan's decision or overturns all or some of the plan's decision. The plan must accept this decision.

Family and Medical Leave Act (FMLA): A federal law that guarantees up to 12 weeks of job protected leave for certain employees when they need to take time off due to serious illness or disability, to have or adopt a child, or to care for another family member. When on leave under FMLA, you can continue coverage under your job-based plan.

Fee for Service: A method in which doctors and other health care providers are paid for each service performed. Examples of services include tests and office visits.

Flexible Benefits Plan: A benefit program that offers employees a choice between various benefits including cash, life insurance, health insurance, vacations, retirement plans, and childcare. Although a common core of benefits may be required, you can choose how your remaining benefit dollars are to be allocated for each type of benefit from the total amount promised by the employer. Sometimes you can contribute more for additional coverage. Also known as a Cafeteria plan or IRS 125 Plan.

Flexible Spending Account (FSA): An arrangement through your employer that lets you pay for many out-of-pocket medical expenses with tax-free dollars. Allowed expenses include insurance co-payments and deductibles, qualified prescription drugs, insulin, and medical devices. You decide how much to put in an FSA, up to a limit set by your employer. You aren't taxed on this money.

- If money is left at the end of the year, the employer can offer one of two options (not both): You get 2.5 more months to spend the leftover money OR you can carry over up to $500 to spend the next plan year.

Formulary: A list of prescription drugs covered by a prescription drug plan or another insurance plan offering prescription drug benefits. Also called a drug list.

Health Maintenance Organization (HMO): A type of health insurance plan that usually limits coverage to care from doctors who work for or contract with the HMO. It generally won't cover out-of-network care except in an emergency. An HMO may require you to live or work in its service area to be eligible for coverage. HMOs often provide integrated care and focus on prevention and wellness.

Health Reimbursement Arrangement (HRA): Health Reimbursement Arrangements (HRAs) are employer-funded group health plans from which employees are reimbursed tax-free for qualified medical expenses up to a fixed dollar amount per year. Unused amounts may be rolled over to be used in subsequent years. The employer funds and owns the arrangement. Health Reimbursement Arrangements are sometimes called Health Reimbursement Accounts.

Health Savings Account (HAS): A type of savings account that lets you set aside money on a pre-tax basis to pay for qualified medical expenses. By using untaxed dollars in a Health Savings Account (HSA) to pay for deductibles, co-payments, co-insurance, and some other expenses, you may be able to lower your overall health care costs. HSA funds generally may not be used to pay premiums. While you can use the funds in an HSA at any time to pay for qualified medical expenses, you may contribute to an HSA only if you have a High Deductible Health Plan (HDHP) — generally a health plan (including a Marketplace plan) that only covers preventive services before the deductible. HSA funds roll over year to year if you don't spend them. An HSA may earn interest or other earnings, which are not taxable. When you view plans in the Marketplace, you can see if they're "HSA-eligible." Some health insurance companies offer HSAs for their HDHPs. Check with your company. You can also open an HSA through some banks and other financial institutions.

High Deductible Health Plan (HDHP): A plan with a higher deductible than a traditional insurance plan. The monthly premium is usually lower, but you pay more health care costs yourself before the insurance company starts to pay its share (your deductible). A high deductible plan (HDHP) can be combined with a health savings account (HSA), allowing you to pay for certain medical expenses with money free from federal taxes.

Home and Community Based Services (HCBS): Services and support provided by most state Medicaid programs in your home or community that gives help with such daily tasks as bathing or dressing. This care is covered when provided by care workers or, if your state permits it, by your family.

Hospital Readmissions: A situation where you were discharged from the hospital and wind up going back in for the same or related care within 30, 60 or 90 days. The number of hospital readmissions is often used in part to measure the quality of hospital care, since it can mean that your follow-up care wasn't properly organized, or that you weren't fully treated before discharge.

Individual Coverage Health Reimbursement Arrangement: A type of Health Reimbursement Arrangement that reimburses medical expenses, like monthly premiums, and requires eligible employees and dependents to have individual health insurance coverage or Medicare Parts A (Hospital Insurance) and B (Medical Insurance) or Part C (Medicare Advantage) for each month they are covered by the individual coverage HRA. An employer can offer an individual coverage HRA instead of other job-based insurance that meets requirements for affordability and minimum value standards. Employees and dependents with an individual coverage HRA offer qualify for premium tax credits only if the employer's offer doesn't meet minimum standards for affordability, and they opt out of individual coverage HRA coverage.

Insurance Co-op: A non-profit entity in which the same people who own the company are insured by the company. Cooperatives can be formed at a national, state or local level, and can include doctors, hospitals and businesses as member-owners.

Medical Underwriting: A process used by insurance companies to try to figure out your health status when you're applying for health insurance coverage to determine whether to offer you coverage, at what price, and with what exclusions or limits.

Medicare: A federal health insurance program for people 65 and older and certain younger people with disabilities. It also covers people with End-Stage Renal Disease (permanent kidney failure requiring dialysis or a transplant, sometimes called ESRD).

Medicare Advantage (Medicare Part C): A type of Medicare health plan offered by a private company that contracts with Medicare to provide you with all your Part A and Part B benefits. Medicare Advantage Plans include Health Maintenance Organizations, Preferred Provider Organizations, Private Fee-for-Service Plans, Special Needs Plans, and Medicare Medical Savings Account Plans. If you're enrolled in a Medicare Advantage Plan, most Medicare services are covered through the plan and aren't paid for under Original Medicare. Most Medicare Advantage Plans offer prescription drug coverage.

Medicare Part D: A program that helps pay for prescription drugs for people with Medicare who join a plan that includes Medicare prescription drug coverage. There are two ways to get Medicare prescription drug coverage: through a Medicare Prescription Drug Plan or a Medicare Advantage Plan that includes drug coverage. These plans are offered by insurance companies and other private companies approved by Medicare.

Open Enrollment Period: The yearly period (November 1 – January 15) when people can enroll in a Marketplace health insurance plan. Outside Open Enrollment, you may still be able to enroll in a Marketplace coverage if you have certain life events, like getting married, having a baby, or losing other health coverage, or based on your estimated household income. Job-based plans may have different Open Enrollment Periods. Check with your employer. You can apply and enroll in Medicaid or the Children's Health Insurance Program (CHIP) any time of year.

Patient Protection and Affordable Care Act: The first part of the comprehensive health care reform law enacted on March 23, 2010. The law was amended by the Health Care and Education Reconciliation Act on March 30, 2010. The name "Affordable Care Act" is usually used to refer to the final, amended version of the law. (It's sometimes known as "PPACA," "ACA," or "Obamacare.") The law provides numerous rights and protections that make health coverage fairer and easier to understand, along with subsidies (through "premium tax credits" and "cost-sharing reductions") to make it more affordable. The law also expands the Medicaid program to cover more people with low incomes.

Payment Bundling: A payment structure in which different health care providers who are treating you for the same or related conditions are paid an overall sum for taking care of your condition rather than being paid for each individual treatment, test, or procedure. In doing so, providers are rewarded for coordinating care, preventing complications and errors, and reducing unnecessary or duplicative tests and treatments.

Point of Service (POS) Plans: A type of plan in which you pay less if you use doctors, hospitals, and other health care providers that belong to the plan's network. POS plans also require you to get a referral from your primary care doctor in order to see a specialist.

Pre-existing Condition: A health problem, like asthma, diabetes, or cancer, you had before the date that new health coverage starts. Insurance companies can't refuse to cover treatment for your pre-existing condition or charge you more.

Pre-existing Condition Exclusion Period (individual policy): The time period during which an individual policy won't pay for care relating to a pre-existing condition. Under an individual policy, conditions may be excluded permanently (known as an "exclusionary rider"). Rules on pre-existing condition exclusion periods in individual policies vary widely by state.

Preauthorization: A decision by your health insurer or plan that a health care service, treatment plan, prescription drug or durable medical equipment is medically necessary. Sometimes called prior authorization, prior approval or precertification. Your health insurance or plan may require preauthorization for certain services before you receive them, except in an emergency. Preauthorization isn't a promise your health insurance or plan will cover the cost.

Preferred Provider: A provider who has a contract with your health insurer or plan to provide services to you at a discount. Check your policy to see if you can see all preferred providers or if your health insurance or plan has a "tiered" network and you must pay extra to see some providers. Your health insurance or plan may have preferred providers who are also "participating" providers. Participating providers also contract with your health insurer or plan, but the discount may not be as great, and you may have to pay more.

Preferred Provider Organization (PPO): A type of health plan that contracts with medical providers, such as hospitals and doctors, to create a network of participating providers. You pay less if you use providers that belong to the plan's network. You can use doctors, hospitals, and providers outside of the network for an additional cost.

Premium: The amount you pay for your health insurance every month. In addition to your premium, you usually have to pay other costs for your health care, including a deductible, co-payments, and co-insurance. If you have a Marketplace health plan, you may be able to lower your costs with a premium tax credit. When shopping for a plan, keep in mind that the plan with the lowest monthly premium may not be the best match for you. If you need a lot of health care, a plan with a slightly higher premium but a lower deductible may save you a lot of money. After you enroll in a plan, you must pay your first premium directly to the insurance company — not to the Health Insurance Marketplace˙.

Preventive Services: Routine health care that includes screenings, check-ups, and patient counseling to prevent illnesses, disease, or other health problems.

Primary Care: Health services that cover a range of prevention, wellness, and treatment for common illnesses. Primary care providers include doctors, nurses, nurse practitioners, and physician assistants. They often maintain long-term relationships with you and advise and treat you on a range of health- related issues. They may also coordinate your care with specialists.

Prior Authorization: Approval from a health plan that may be required before you get a service or fill a prescription in order for that service or prescription to be covered by your plan.

Qualified Health Plan: An insurance plan that's certified by the Health Insurance Marketplace˙, provides essential health benefits, follows established limits on cost-sharing (like deductibles, copayments, and out-of-pocket maximum amounts), and meets other requirements under the Affordable Care Act. All qualified health plans meet the Affordable Care Act requirement for having health coverage, known as "minimum essential coverage."

Qualifying Life Event (QLE): A change in your situation — like getting married, having a baby, or losing health coverage — that can make you eligible for a Special Enrollment Period, allowing you to enroll in health insurance outside the yearly Open Enrollment Period.

Referral: A written order from your primary care doctor for you to see a specialist or get certain medical services. In many Health Maintenance Organizations (HMOs), you need to get a referral before you can get medical care from anyone except your primary care doctor. If you don't get a referral first, the plan may not pay for the services.

Rider: A rider is an amendment to an insurance policy. Some riders add coverage (for example, if you buy a maternity rider to add coverage for pregnancy to your policy).

Risk Adjustment: A statistical process that takes into account the underlying health status and health spending of the enrollees in an insurance plan when looking at their health care outcomes or health care costs.

Self-Insured Plans: Type of plan that is usually present in larger companies where the employer itself collects premiums from enrollees and takes on the responsibility of paying employees' and dependents' medical claims. These employers can contract for insurance services such as enrollment, claims processing, and provider networks with a third-party administrator, or they can be self-administered.

Skilled Nursing Care: Services from licensed nurses in your own home or in a nursing home. Skilled care services are from technicians and therapists in your own home or in a nursing home.

Skilled Nursing Facility Care: Skilled nursing care and rehabilitation services provided on a continuous, daily basis in a skilled nursing facility. Examples of skilled nursing facility care include physical therapy or intravenous injections that can only be given by a registered nurse or doctor.

Special Enrollment Period: A time outside the yearly Open Enrollment Period when you can sign up for health insurance. You qualify for a Special Enrollment Period if you've had certain life events, including losing health coverage, moving, getting married, having a baby, or adopting a child, or if your household income is below a certain amount. Depending on your Special Enrollment Period type, you may have 60 days before or 60 days following the event to enroll in a plan. You can enroll in Medicaid or the Children's Health Insurance

Program (CHIP) any time. Job-based plans must provide a Special Enrollment Period of at least 30 days.

Specialist: A physician specialist focuses on a specific area of medicine or a group of patients to diagnose, manage, prevent or treat certain types of symptoms and conditions. A non-physician specialist is a provider who has more training in a specific area of health care.

Subsidized Coverage: Health coverage available at reduced or no cost for people with incomes below certain levels. Examples of subsidized coverage include Medicaid and the Children's Health Insurance Program (CHIP). Marketplace insurance plans with premium tax credits are sometimes known as subsidized coverage too.

UCR (usual, customary and reasonable): The amount paid for a medical service in a geographic area based on what providers in the area usually charge for the same or similar medical service. The UCR amount sometimes is used to determine the allowed amount.

Uncompensated Care: Health care or services provided by hospitals or health care providers that don't get reimbursed. Often uncompensated care arises when people don't have insurance and cannot afford to pay the cost of care.

Value Based Purchasing (VBP): Linking provider payments to improved performance by health care providers. This form of payment holds health care providers accountable for both the cost and quality of care they provide. It attempts to reduce inappropriate care and to identify and reward the best-performing providers.

Well-baby and Well-child Visits: Routine doctor visits for comprehensive preventive health services that occur when a baby is young and annual visits until a child reaches age 21. Services include physical exam and measurements, vision and hearing screening, and oral health risk assessments.

Wellness Program: A program intended to improve and promote health and fitness that's usually offered through the workplace, although insurance plans can offer them directly to their enrollees. The program allows your employer or plan to offer you premium discounts, cash rewards, gym memberships, and other incentives to participate. Some examples of wellness programs include programs to help you stop smoking, diabetes management programs, weight loss programs, and preventative health screenings.

About the Author

Amy Fitzgerald Pelloquin grew up in Louisiana and spent much of her early years as a physician in the South. She initially worked at an academic medical center teaching, writing, lecturing and seeing patients in primary care. As her children grew, so did the demands of academics, so she transitioned to private practice where she worked for many years. She then branched out into Integrative Medicine and has never looked back. She believes that disease is a manifestation of disharmony in the body on multiple levels and is always looking for innovative non-traditional ways that people can support their own health.

She currently lives in Colorado with her husband and dogs, and enjoys hiking, cooking, writing, communing with the mountains and spending as much time outdoors as possible.

WHAT I WISH MY PATIENTS MY KNEW...